Meal Prep

Low Carb Weight Loss Recipes

Table of Contents

Introduction 7

Chapter 1: Why Should We Do Meal Preps? 10

Chapter 2: How to Get Started with Meal Prep? 24

Chapter 3: How to Prep for a Low Carb Diet? 39

Chapter 4: Important Steps for Meal Prep 44

Chapter 5: How to Have Fun with Meal Preps 55

Chapter 6: Breakfast Recipes 60

    Chocolate Peanut Butter Cups 60

    Baked Oatmeal Cups with Raisins and Walnuts 62

    Coconut Carrot Morning Glory Muffins 64

    Green Muffins 66

    Tofu Scramble & Breakfast Sweet Potatoes 68

    Potato, Asparagus & Mushroom Hash 70

    Vegan Omelet 72

    Breakfast Burritos 74

    Spinach and Broccoli Strata 76

Prosciutto & Asparagus Strata 78

Pumpkin Pancakes 81

Chapter 7: Snack Recipes 83

Monkey Cookies... 83

Ham, Swiss, and Spinach Roll Ups 84

Tri-berry Yogurt Pops.. 85

Baked Parmesan Fries 86

Guacamole Devilled Eggs 87

Easy Baked Parmesan Mushrooms 88

Citrus Chicken Salad Strips 89

Maple Chai Roasted Chickpeas 91

Honey Nut Granola... 92

Parmesan Carrot Fries 93

Asian Turkey Lettuce Wraps 94

Healthy Cookie Dough Peanut Butter Protein Balls 96

Sweet Potato Hummus 97

White Bean and Roasted Red Pepper Hummus 98

Mini Peanut Butter and Apple Sandwich............................. 99

Broccoli Parmesan Meatballs 101

Chapter 8: Lunch Recipes 103

Chicken and Black Bean Burrito Salad in a Mason jar 103

BLT Pasta Salad 105

Greek Courgetti Salad 106

Griddled Salad Jar 107

Creamy Radish Soup... 109

Carrot and Ginger Immune Boosting Soup...................... 111

Green Soup with Chicken 112

Turkey and Spring Onion Wraps...................................... 114

Carrot and Hummus Roll Ups 115

Prawn Sweet Chili Noodle Salad 116

Vegetarian Reuben with Russian dressing...................... 118

Sesame Noodles 120

Maple Roasted Sweet Potatoes.. 122

Easy Pasta Salad 123

Chapter 9: Dinner Recipes 124

Miso Noodle Soup... 124

Chickpea and Sausage Pesto Soup................................... 126

Split Pea Soup 127

Vegan Chili 129

Sweet Potato Casserole 131

Classic Dinner Pancakes 133

Potato Rounds with Fresh Lemon 135

Baked Mac & Cheese 136

Bacon Turkey Burger 138

Southwestern Cheddar Steak Fries 140

Oven Baked Chicken Strips 142

Mediterranean Chicken Quinoa Bowl 143

Buffalo Chicken Casserole 145

Smoky Beef Stew 147

Spicy Smoky Sweet Chili 148

Steak Burritos 150

Sole en Papillotte 152

Quick Shrimp Enchilada Bake 153

Skillet Tuna Noodle Casserole 155

Middle Eastern Lamb Stew 157

Conclusion 159

© Copyright 2018 - All rights reserved.

The contents of this book may not be reproduced, duplicated or transmitted without direct written permission from the author.

Under no circumstances will any legal responsibility or blame be held against the publisher for any reparation, damages, or monetary loss due to the information herein, either directly or indirectly.

Legal Notice:

This book is copyright protected. This is only for personal use. You cannot amend, distribute, sell, use, quote or paraphrase any part or the content within this book without the consent of the author.

Disclaimer Notice:

Please note the information contained within this document is for educational and entertainment purposes only. Every attempt has been made to provide accurate, up to date and reliable complete information. No warranties of any kind are expressed or implied. Readers acknowledge that the author is not engaging in the rendering of legal, financial, medical or professional advice. The content of this book has been derived from various sources. Please consult a licensed professional before attempting any techniques outlined in this book.

The trademarks that are used are without any consent, and the publication of the trademark is without permission or backing by the trademark owner. All trademarks and brands within this book are for clarifying purposes only and are owned by the owners themselves, not affiliated with this document.

By reading this document, the reader agrees that under no circumstances are is the author responsible for any losses, direct or indirect, which are incurred as result of the use of information contained within this document, including, but not limited to errors, omissions, or inaccuracies.

Introduction

Thank you for choosing this book, 'Meal Prep – The Lazy Low Carb Weight Loss Recipes.'

Do you often feel irritated at the thought of having to cook your meals after a long day's work? Well, here's good news for you. You no longer have to go through the grueling process of putting together last-minute meals. I am so excited to share a simple, yet effective way of revolutionizing your kitchen life through meal planning. I am sincerely hoping that this guide acts as a catalyst for change when it comes to preparing your meals. Through this book, you will not only discover the joy of relishing a simple yet delicious meal with your family but also be able to enjoy a relaxed cooking experience. Within no time you will become an expert in whipping up some mouth-watering dishes quickly. You will also be able to pass on the knowledge to many others like you who wish to learn the art of meal planning.

As people from the 21st century, many of us haven't received a lot of training to do with budgeting for food, making a shopping list, picking the best ingredients from the market and learning how to use leftovers. However, the art of meal preparation is not rocket science. Even if you are a beginner, you can choose to whip up some simple and healthy recipes without much help. Eating out frequently without paying much attention to nutrition can weaken our body's immune system over a period. Of course, we may not notice any symptom right now, but if we were to continue leading an unhealthy lifestyle, we can be vulnerable to developing various kinds of chronic illnesses.

Before I started prepping for meals, I always preferred just throwing whatever ingredients I got my hands on into the cooker and preparing some basic dishes. Just the fact that I was making sure that my family was eating home cooked meals, instead of outside food, was enough for me to feel satisfied with my cooking style. I soon started realizing how almost everyone in the family had started making excuses to not eat my home cooked meals.

I too couldn't stick to the low carb diet I had recently taken up. After all, how could someone keep on eating the same boring food repeatedly days over days? At that time, meal prepping seemed like an excellent idea, where I could organize what I eat, what ingredients I use and even control my portions. Initially, I thought I would not be able to keep up with the meal prep plan, but merely within a week, I was able to handle it just fine. Ever since, I feel relaxed and have a great time while cooking my meals.

I am hoping that this guide can help you with all the essential information you need to know about meal prepping and more. In this book, there are a good list of easy and lip-smacking recipes that help you get started and make your meal preps more fun. Keep reading to find out more!

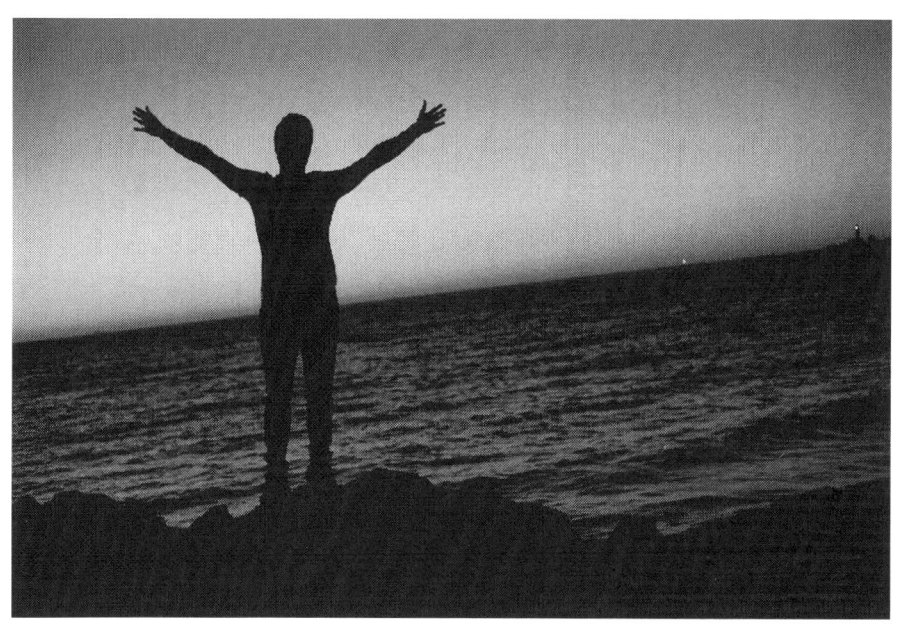

Chapter 1: Why Should We Do Meal Preps?

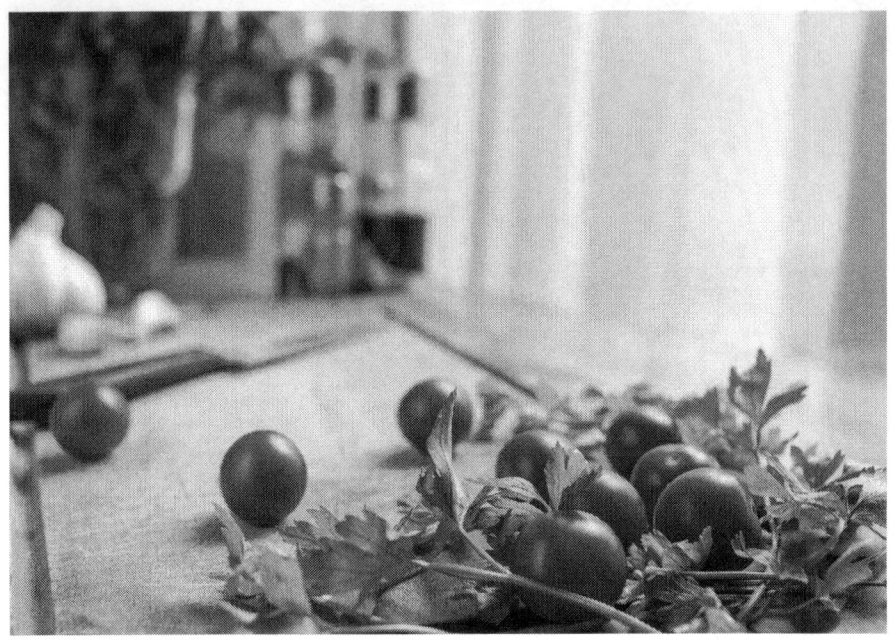

If you think meal preps are unnecessary, and you can completely do without it, you are about to discover how wrong you are. The fact is if you are doing any kind of home-made meals, you are already doing some form of meal prep. To many who have not tried meal prep in more efficient scale, meal planning may sound like it's immensely time consuming and that it just adds up to your daily chores, but that's not true. In fact, once you get good at meal prepping, you will realize how much easier your life will get. If you have a busy schedule, then it's even more vital that you spend some time planning your meals. When you prepare well ahead for your meals, you are going to be able to make the most of your day to accomplish everything you want to. We don't realize the amount of time we waste on cooking our meals haphazardly when we could be utilizing the same time to focus on various other activities. Meal preps allow you the time to unwind after having had a long day. Once you start organizing your meals, you will experience the satisfactory feeling of having a perfectly executed day. Let's look at how meal preps can help you with your day-to-day life.

Saves Time

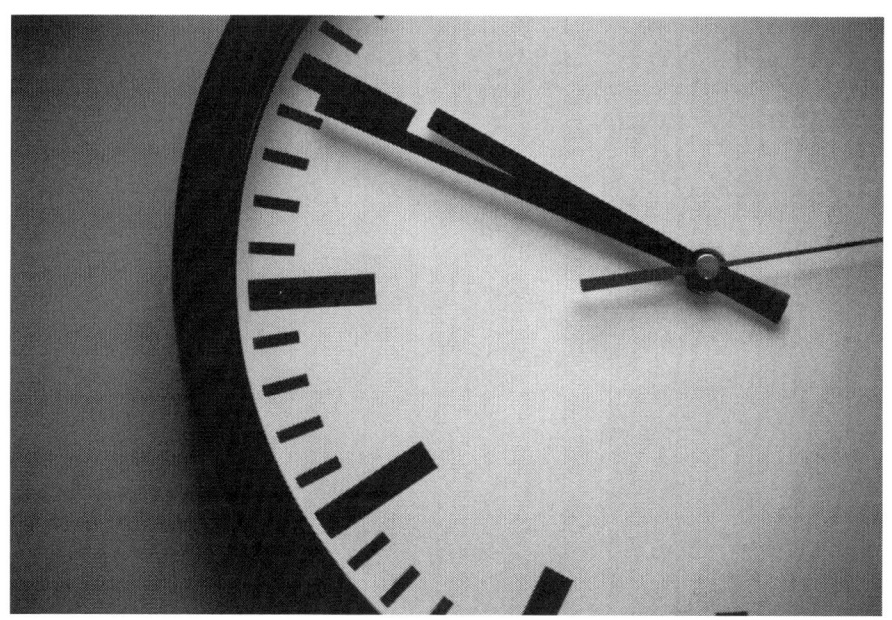

Those frequent errands you make to fetch groceries or to whip up your meals in a hurry is not only energy draining but also consumes a lot of your precious time. It also makes you more anxious, and even though you may be great cook otherwise, you end up making some mediocre dishes for your family. I know it's hard to imagine that prepping up for your meals for an entire week may help you in saving any time, but it does. You may have cooked large meals before, and you may think prepping's no big deal, however, you will soon notice how you end up saving hours of hard work. Imagine having to spend just about half the time you require to cook dinner for your family. Also, don't we all hate cleaning up after the meals? To avoid this, meal prepping can help you plan one or two large meals in a week; thereby saving the time you spend on clean ups.

Saves Money

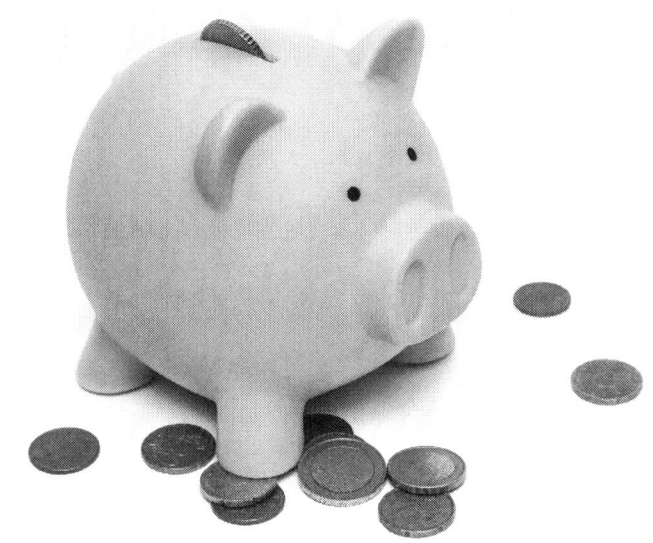

Sure, the newly opened local restaurants offer a variety of dishes and that are at low prices. So, you head towards one of these outlets almost every single day to have some snacks or meals. You may not realize, but those daily expenses can end up drilling a hole in your pocket. It's only when you start tracking your expenses that you realize how much extra money you are spending on outside food. When you eat out, you are not only paying for the dish, but you are also paying for the labor, the décor, and even the gas used for preparing the food. So how about cutting down all those expenses by cooking at home with minimal planning? All you have to do is buy some fresh produce for the entire week and whip up some easy recipes. This can drastically reduce your monthly expenses.

Helps Control Nutrition in Your Meals

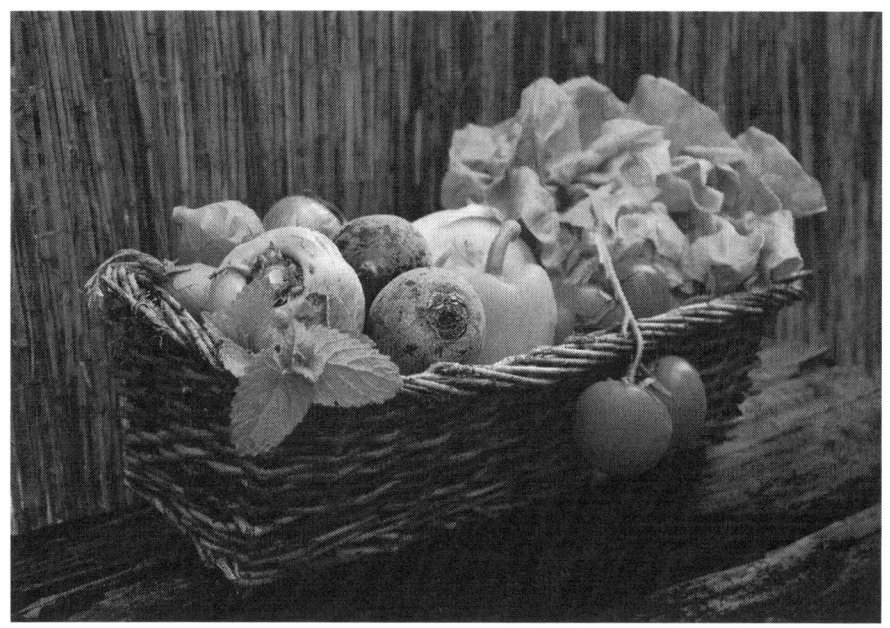

Unlike the restaurant food, when you prepare meals at home, you can choose not to add excess salt, sugar, oil or MSG. Similarly, you can also control the protein, fats and carbohydrate portion in your daily intake. From various studies, we are prone to eating whatever is in front of us without realizing the excess calories we ingest. While prepping up your meals, you can store the food in a pre-portioned container, so you don't end up overeating. There are numerous times when we are compelled to cook a dinner from scratch after a tiring day, and we end up consuming unhealthier options. When you start preparing healthier meals at home, you can better control the nutrition in your food, and thereby drop a lot of body fat too.

Stress Relief

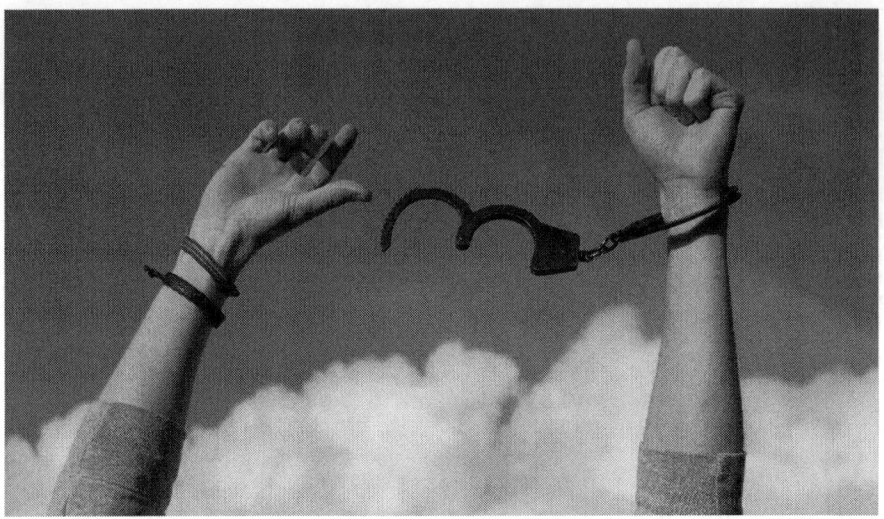

Are you someone who always multitasks and end up stressing yourself out for a meal? Last-minute meals require a lot of time and energy. They make you race home from a long day and get everything done within a short period. The result? Tasteless food and a lot of exhaustion! Is it worth all the hassle? Why not just spend some time prepping up for your dinner a little ahead and have a more relaxed time? When you have a meal plan, you are less likely to run out of time, and that can make you want to whip even tastier food. Meal preps will make you want to eagerly look forward to coming home to an easy and delicious dinner.

Makes Shopping Easier

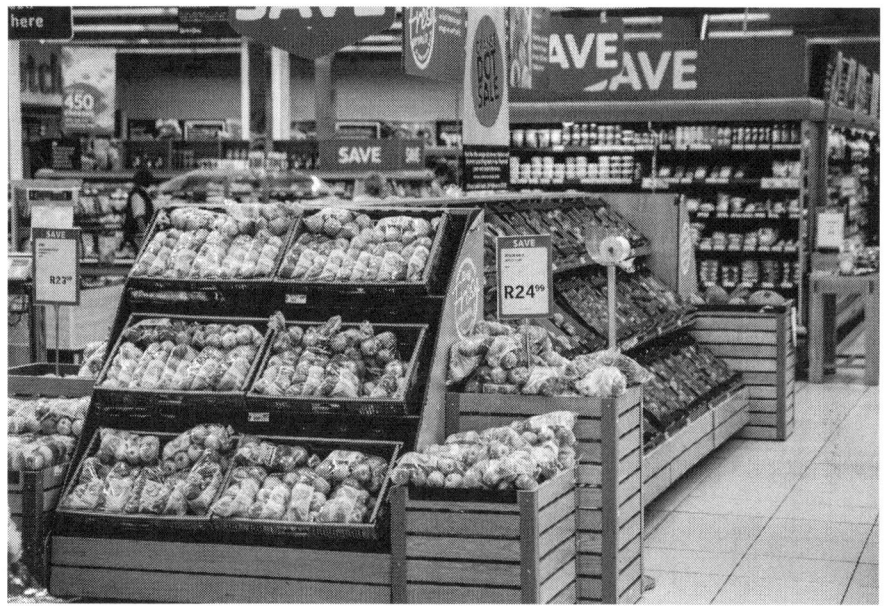

When we run last minute errands to the grocery shop, we end up paying more for those smaller packets of ingredients, not to mention the amount of stress it brings to squeeze in time from your busy work schedule to make a trip to the supermarket. On the other hand, when you prepare a list of things to buy for the entire month, you are less likely to run out of the ingredients. It will help you carefully analyze the items that you need to buy in larger quantities, so you don't have to visit the supermarket so frequently. The next time you are out to do some grocery shopping, I bet you will be having some fun too.

Tastier Meals

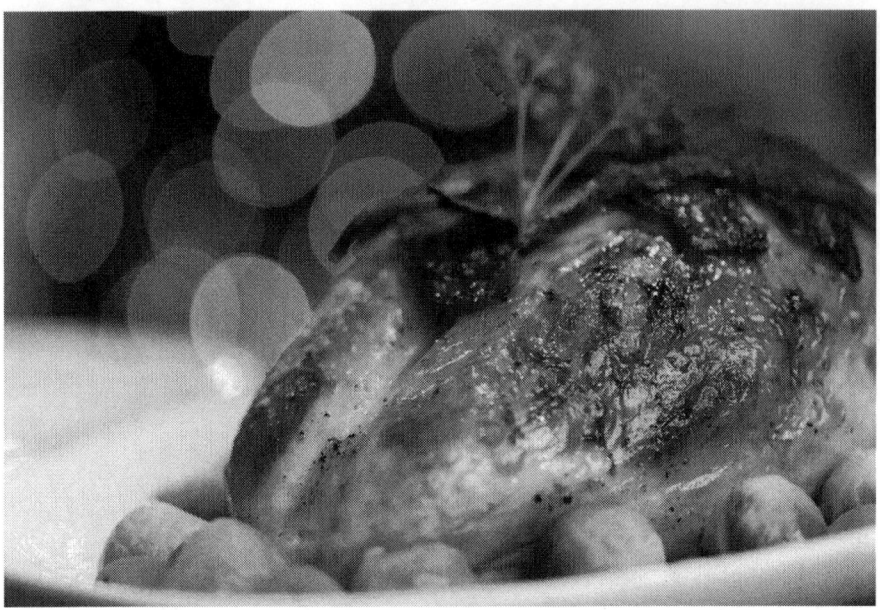

How often have you just thrown all the ingredients in your pan and cooked up a mediocre dish? If this has been happening a lot, it's likely that you aren't preparing for your meals. Not prepping up for your meals may prevent you from making tastier meals for your family. When you run out of ingredients or time for preparing your meals, it automatically undermines your cooking skills. To be able to cook tastier meals, you need to put some thought into how you want it to turn out and accordingly keep the ingredients ready. Planned meals also allow you to assess how time you would be able to spare for making each dish, thus avoiding disappointment.

Prevents Food Wastage

When prepping for your meals, you familiarize yourself with the inventory of ingredients in your kitchen. Keeping a record of what you already have in your kitchen and what it is that you need, helps in keeping us accountable for wastage. Also, when you organize your meals, you may end up utilizing that half a lemon or those kale leaves lying around in your fridge. You are less likely to waste leftovers and more likely to include them while making pasta, burrito bowls or even salads. You can also store some ingredients in airtight containers and label them, so you don't forget to use them while cooking. Meal prepping helps you identify how much food you are wasting, and eventually helps you become more careful about how you utilize almost about everything in your kitchen.

Food Variety

Until a couple of years ago, I would only cook broccoli and bananas for breakfast because I considered them super nutritious. Of course, they are, but I stuck to those ingredients also out of convenience. They were readily available and hence buying them wasn't a hassle. Although my family loves bananas and broccoli, they soon started to loathe the sight of it, so much so that they refused to eat anything that had these two ingredients in it. Bottom line, don't stick to limited ingredients just because they are nutritious, your body needs a variety of vitamins, minerals as well as nutritious to function well.

When you put some thought into making your meals, you tend to choose several different types of ingredients instead of only sticking to the ones you would buy. This helps in breaking the monotony of your meals and makes you want to look forward to every meal. Once you start having different kinds of ingredients, you can easily put together a great meal.

You Make Fewer Snap Decisions

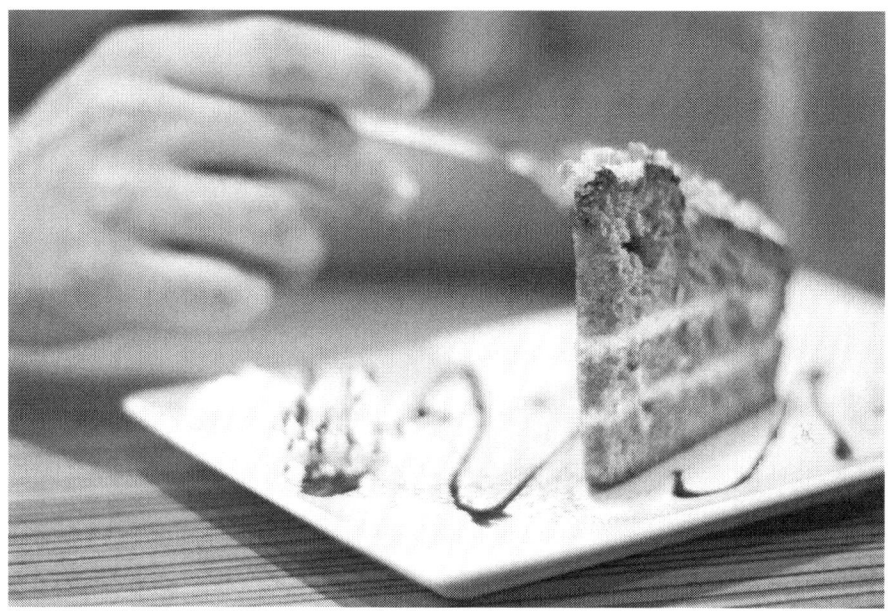

Even the most self-disciplined person would be tempted to give in when hunger pangs come calling. When your stomach starts growling, you tend to be more prone to cravings, and chances are that you may not pick the healthiest of ingredients when this happens. Such cravings will not just be expensive for your wallet, but they can also throw you off from your diet plan. By prepping up for your entire week or month's meals, you turn something that's instinctual into cerebral. You should never hit the grocery shop when you are most hungry. Moreover, avoid circumstances that make you want to rush to the grocery shop by preparing your meals ahead. Do not let your body choose meals for you; you choose the meals for your body.

Teaches Portion Control

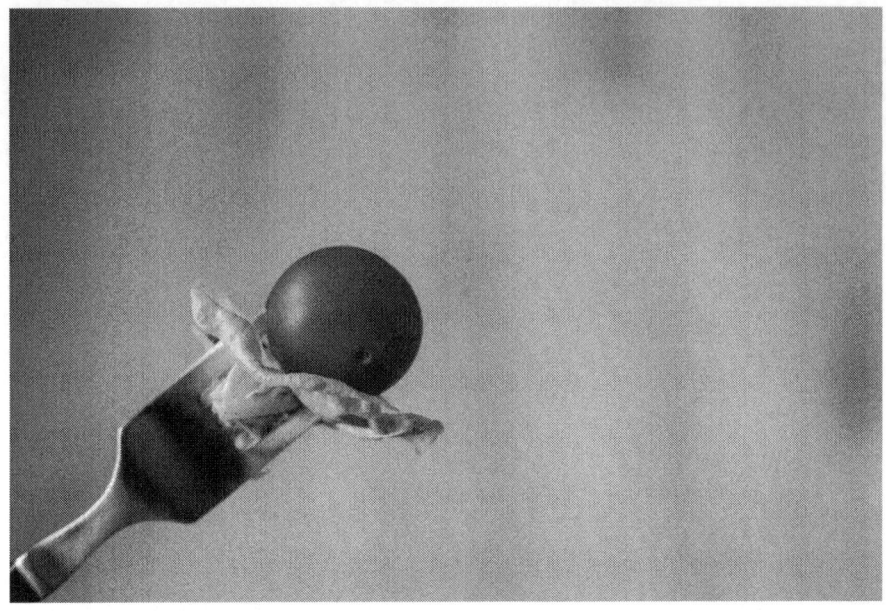

Self-control is not just about eating right; it's also about eating in the right quantities. You can always enjoy family style dinners on Sundays, but weekday meals packed in containers in allotted portions can teach you a thing or two about portion control. Regardless of whether you're trying to lose weight or attempting to gain muscle, keeping track of your food portions is extremely vital. When you don't think about your food portions, you will almost always end up overeating, thereby consuming additional calories. Meal prep, on the other hand, keeps your food intake balanced. When you pack your meals in Tupperware containers while eating only an allotted portion, your body learns to discipline itself. You can certainly indulge in occasional treats, but when you become wiser about your food intake, you are less likely to lose control.

Chapter 2: How to Get Started with Meal Prep?

In this chapter, you are going to learn the easiest version of meal prep, which will successfully get you started. If you have never prepped for your meals, now is the time to give it a serious thought. Accomplishing this meal prep plan almost every week can offer your enormous help in your day-to-day life. Prepping up for your meal isn't as time-consuming as you think, except if you waste too much time thinking rather than getting into action. If you are making a meal plan for the very first time, you may need some help. However, once you get into the groove, meal preps will not only become easier, but they will seem a lot of fun too.

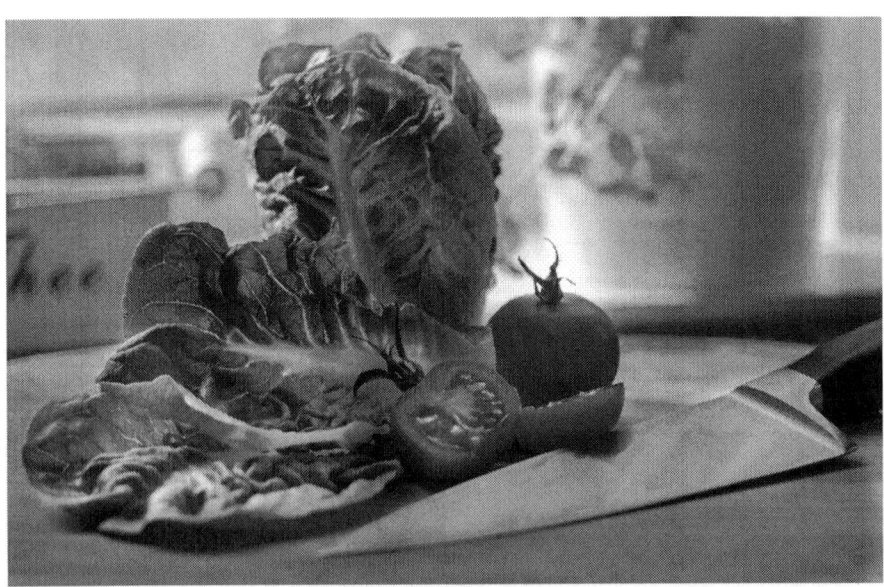

So, let's quickly get to it. You can choose to prep for daily, weekly or even monthly meals. Everyone works on a different schedule, so you can feel free to pick a plan of your choice. But if you have a busy schedule, it is recommended that you plan a week ahead. The basic idea is to start sorting out the smallest of things and be patient with yourself while you are chalking out your meal plans.

Cleaning Up Your Kitchen

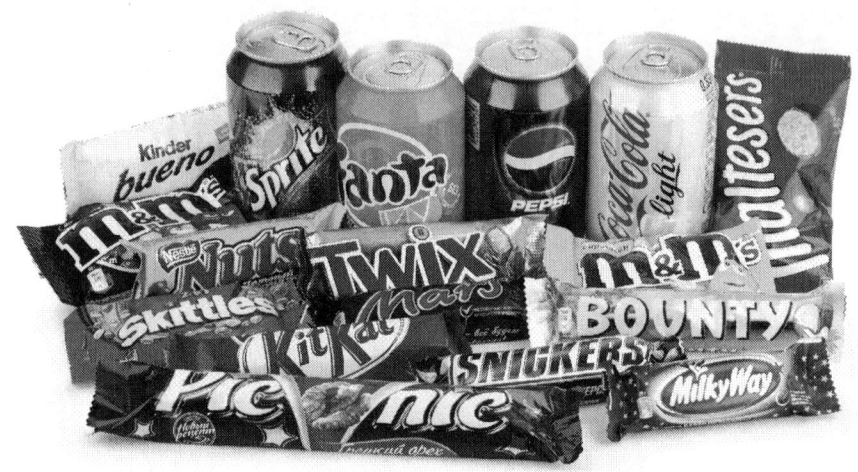

This is very important especially if you are going on a weight loss diet. The "Out of sight is out of mind" mantra would immensely benefit someone who is trying to lose weight while their kitchen is stocked with all kind of unhealthy items. So you start by literally throwing away the junk food or giving it away to the homeless. Next, start cleaning up your kitchen and gather some Tupperware containers because you are going to need them a lot once you start your meal preps. Ensure that you leave a lot of space in the kitchen as you are going to stack it up with ingredients for the entire week.

Food Storage

When it comes to food storage, you need to find the right containers. These containers will be used for storing all kinds of ingredients and sometimes even cooked meals in allotted portions. So it's important that you store food in containers that are completely safe and easy to clean. Following are the things that you need to consider while picking the containers for your meal plans.

- Imagine packing a liquid meal in a container and carrying it in your bag only to find out that the food has spilled all over it. Extremely frustrating. I agree. If you are going to store liquids, you are going to need airtight and leak-proof lids. A good lid will not only prevent leakage but also keep the food fresh. To test a new container, fill it with some liquid, close the lid and shake it a few times to check if it's leaking or the lid accidentally opens up. Try dropping in something hot and notice if it cracks or the lid stays on.

- We all like to eat straight out of containers sometimes. After all, it's convenient, right? Except the fact that some containers or their lids aren't made of a material that allows it to be used in a microwave. If you are not aware of this, you may end up contributing towards some serious health concerns. Melted plastic is extremely hazardous for our bodies in the long run.

- Pick containers that can easily fit into your bag while you are traveling. Lightweight, sleek and portable containers should be a meal prep expert's best friend. There are various types of containers available in the market, some with a single compartment and the other with multiple compartments. You can pick one as per your needs.

Condiments and Spices

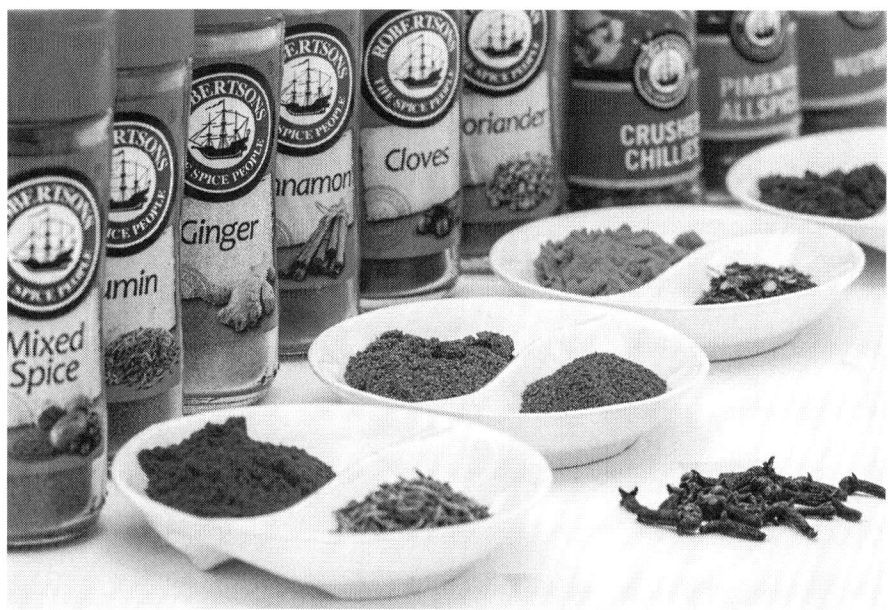

So you have decided to eat healthier meals, but they don't have to be tasteless. You are going need a lot of condiments and spices if you to add some great flavor to your meals. Spices and seasonings can instantly enhance the flavors of any dish and help you reap some health benefits too. Hence, the next time you prep for meals, don't forget to add a lot of them. Some of these essential spices and condiments you are going to need are mentioned as following.

Turmeric

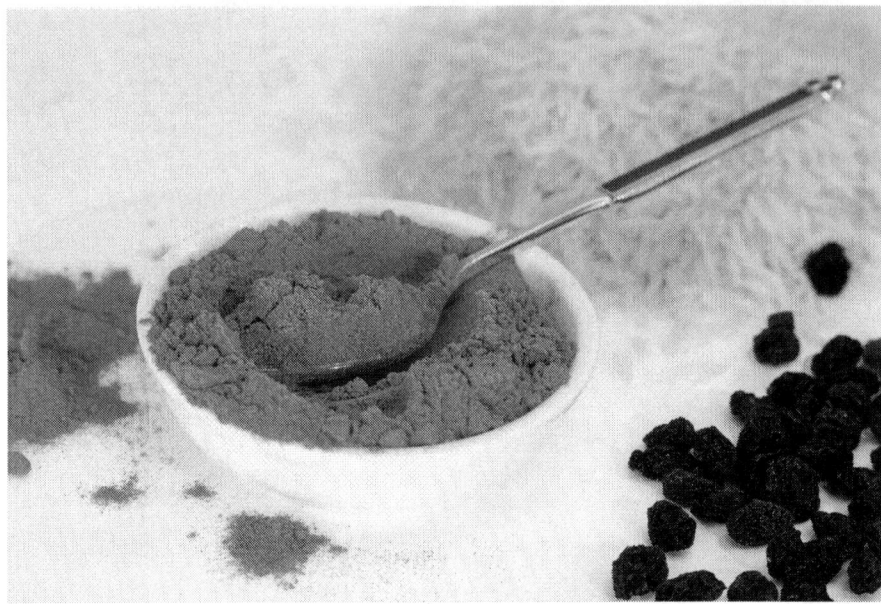

This Indian spice not only adds a beautiful flavor to your food but offers a lot of health benefits too. It helps your body in creating enzymes that prevent you from storing excess fat and boosts your metabolism. Turmeric also provides various medicinal benefits while protecting you from developing a common cold, fever, and other chronic illnesses.

Himalayan Salt

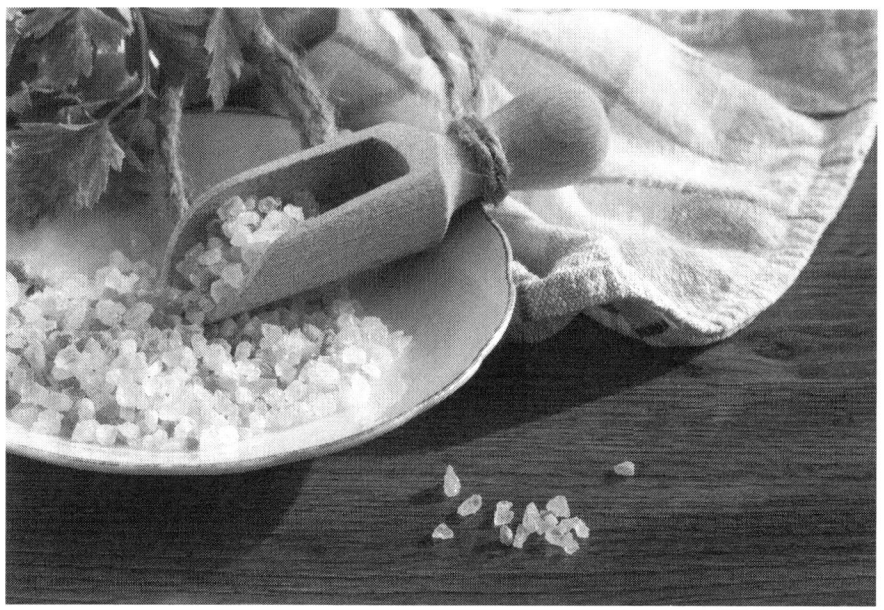

If there is one ingredient with super power qualities, Himalayan salt is your best bet. Unlike other salts that can cause inflammation, blood pressure issues or cardiovascular diseases, Himalayan salt can, in fact, strengthens your immune system. This salt is particularly mined straight from the earth and contains almost 84 minerals that can keep your body healthy. There are studies which showed that people who consumed Himalayan salt demonstrated vast improvement in their respiratory conditions and overall body functions.

Oregano

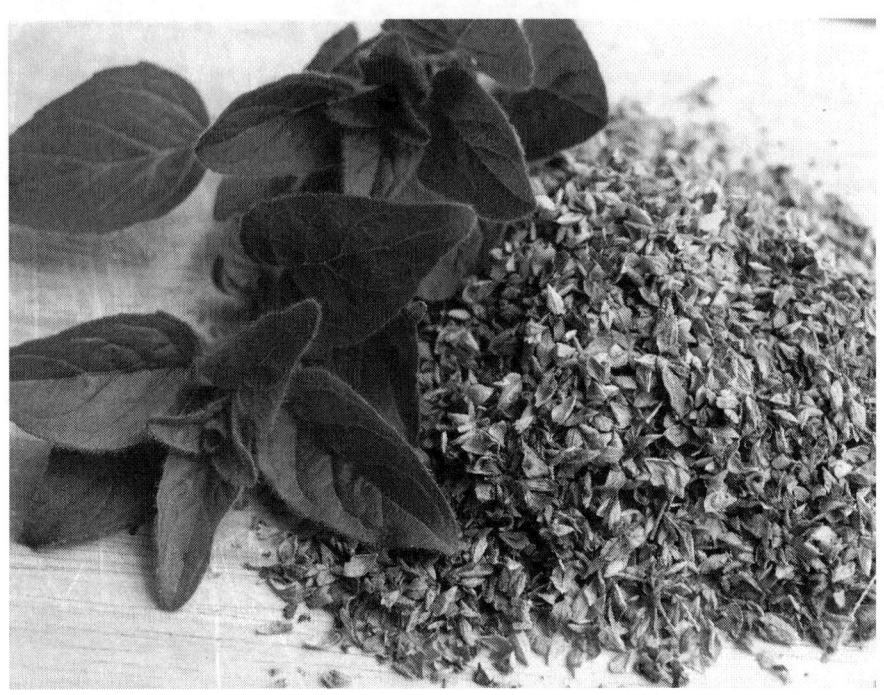

Oregano is known to reduce inflammation and acts as an excellent flavor booster in the food. It can instantly turn a plain dish into a much flavorful one. You can add oregano to pizza, pasta, chicken or even pesto sauce.

Mustard

Add a spoonful of crushed mustard to your next meal and experience the magic of its flavor. Mustard contains certain enzymes that offer cancer-fighting abilities and helps you absorb more nutrients as per a research conducted in "British Journal of Nutrition."

Ketchup

You can buy it from the supermarket or make some at home. Ketchup acts as a handy condiment that can be served along with numerous recipes such as burgers, sandwiches, pizzas, pasta, and rolls. If you choose to buy a bottle of ketchup off the market, make sure it's an organic one.

Mayonnaise

Who doesn't like mayonnaise? Most of us do. You can make various kinds of dips with this condiment that can be served alongside most dishes. You can make low-fat or eggless mayonnaise and store it in an airtight container for use. Similarly, you can also make some vegan mayonnaise by using some Greek yogurt.

Soy Sauce

This is one of the most versatile of all the sauces that can also be added to already-cooked dishes. Soy sauce is not just used for Chinese dishes, but it can also be used for different kinds of salads, soups, and curries too. Depending on your taste preference, you can use light or dark soy sauce to flavor your dishes.

Barbecue Sauce

Almost everyone can easily make barbecue sauce at home. The barbecue sauce recipe requires a blend of tomato puree, a bit of sweetener, spices and an acid. You can adjust the measurements of the ingredients as per your taste. This delicious sauce can be used to make chicken, sandwiched, tempeh ribs, balsamic BBQ, meatballs, tofu wings, etc.

Cooking Equipment

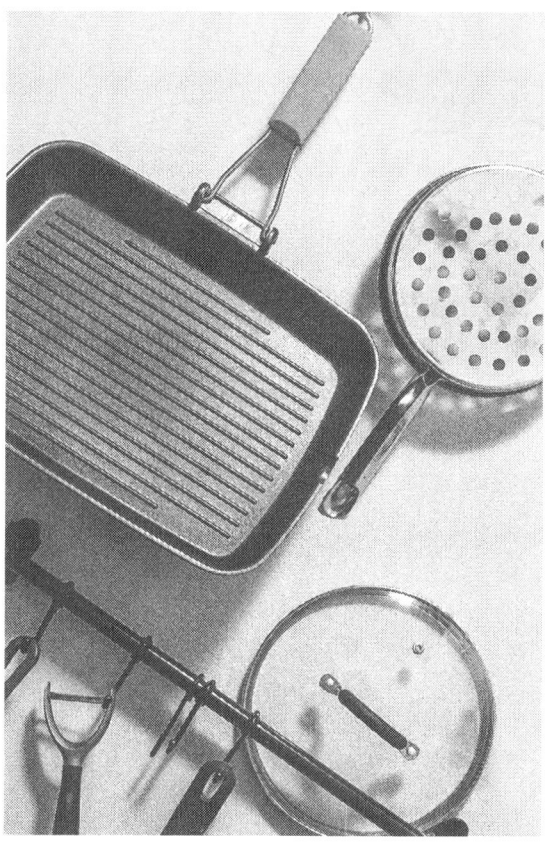

You don't necessarily have to buy any special equipment to start off with your meal-prepping plan. However, having a few tools handy can make your life easier. If you haven't already gathered these tools, waste no more time to get started. Some of this essential cooking equipment is mentioned below.

Slow Cooker

A lot of people think slow cookers are for people who have plenty of time to cook. In fact, slow cookers can be used by the busiest of individuals as you can just dump all the ingredients and go about your work. If you cook the food on low heat, it takes about 6-8 hours, which leaves you with a lot of time to finish your daily chores. Slow cooker meals are generally considered to be tastier as well as healthier. It also allows you to prepare your meals in larger quantities.

Cast Iron Skillet

The timeless cast-iron skillet holds the capacity to produce high heat while retaining it too. This helps in proper searing of protein-rich items such as pork, beef, and chicken. The same skillet can be used to make frittatas, cornbread, deep-dish pizza and stir fry vegetables. A coated skillet can be the best option to cook some delicate food items such as pancakes, omelets and even scrambled eggs.

Food Processor

You may think, "Why do I need a food processor when I have a blender?" The blender certainly does an excellent job of pureeing soups and shakes but struggles while churning nuts or seeds. A food processor can easily pulverize even the toughest of foods in just about a few seconds. The next time you plan to make your energy bars, use the food processor to pulverize some nuts, dry fruits and seeds.

Measuring cups

If you think you don't need them, think again. Measuring cups are essential especially if you like trying out new recipes. If you are an expert and don't need to measure every ingredient you add while making the dish, you will certainly need these measuring cups when you are baking cakes. With the help of these cups, you will never get that amount of baking soda wrong. Accurate measurements always offer consistent results.

Meal Recipes

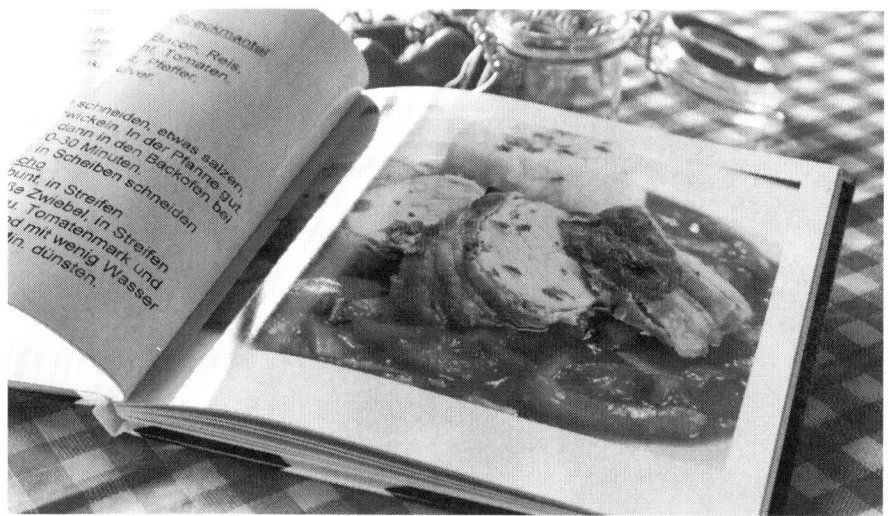

Eating healthier and tastier week after week requires you to be ready with several recipes that can be whipped in no time. After all, you can only have so much scrambled egg and pancakes for breakfast before you need to revamp your meal prep. When you have ample of meal recipes ready, you can turn the standard ingredients such as sweet potato, carrots, broccoli, eggs, bacon chicken, etc. on their heads.

Chapter 3: How to Prep for a Low Carb Diet?

The low carb diet is pretty much designed for everyone, and almost anyone can easily follow it with some knowledge. The amount of carbs you want to consume while on this diet depends on your health goals. It will differ for someone who is trying to lose weight, diabetics or simply trying to lead a healthy lifestyle. A lot of people cringe at the thought of giving up their habit of indulging in unhealthy food items such as cakes, cookies, chocolates, pizzas, fries, etc. All you need to do is do your best to cut down as many unhealthy items from your diet as possible and get closer to your goal with every step. When you start slowly reducing your carbohydrate consumption each day, you will be pleasantly surprised with the weight loss results.

Prepping for low carb diet becomes easier when you know which foods to eat and which ones to avoid. Take a look below.

What can you eat on a low carb diet?
- Meat – Lean meats of all kinds
- Fish – All types of fish, especially the ones high in Omega 3 fatty acids

- Vegetables – Load up on veggies such as spinach, kale, broccoli, cauliflower, avocados, capsicums, mushrooms, lettuce, etc.
- Chicken – free range or skinless
- Cheese – all kinds of cheese
- Cream – Full fat
- Milk – Full fat and all kinds of milk including almond milk, coconut milk, cow's milk, etc.
- Eggs – Preferably organic
- Fruits – Go for low carb fruits such as berries and other citrus fruits
- Fats – Butter, olive oil, coconut oil, etc.

What do you need to avoid on a low carb diet?

- All sugary drinks
- Cakes, biscuits, cookies, pastries, jams
- All kinds of seed oils like sunflower, corn, canola or margarine
- All types of cereals
- Bread, pasta, potatoes, rice
- All types of starchy fruits
- Starchy veggies
- Low-fat products
- All wheat products
- All kinds of grains

How to meal prep for Low carb diet?

Follow the same steps as the above chapter when it comes to meal prepping for a low carb diet. Besides that, remember the amount of proteins, fats and carbohydrates you need to consume. Your daily intakes should contain about 70% of fats, 25% of proteins and about 5% of carbohydrates. You are allowed about 20-30 net carbs each day, but the lower the intake; the better it is for you if you want to reduce body fats. Proteins need to be consumed pretty much every day depending on your needs. For example, if you are looking to bulk up, you may need to take about 1g of protein daily per pound of your body weight. As for your fat intake, it depends on your diet regime that you are following. For instance, Ketogenic and Mediterranean diet often advocate consuming high healthy fats, whereas Paleo diet may not specifically recommend so. As a good general yard stick, always pick healthier fats such as grass-fed butter or cheese over margarine. Mentioned below are a few meal prep tips for low carb ingredients

Proteins

- Always buy organic, or grass-fed meats from the farmer's market.
- Clean the meat properly using paper towels and then pat it dry. You can also slice it up using a sharp knife before storing.

- Wrap the meat with a plastic film and store it in the freezer until you are ready to use it.
- Don't forget to bring the meat to room temperature before you start cooking.
- While cooking meats, you can brown them or braise them before cooking it further. This will help in enhancing the flavor of the dish.

Carbohydrates

- Since you are going to limit your carbohydrate intake, ensure that you add the right portion to your meals.
- Use less starchy veggies for preparing your meals. If you are going to use a lot of vegetables for your meals, wash them properly under running water and pat them dry using paper towels or with a salad spinner. You can chop the veggies using a chef knife and store them in an airtight container.
- Ensure that the vegetables are not moist to avoid them from getting spoiled.
- Sauté them slightly before you cook them for extracting the maximum flavor.
- If you are using other low carb ingredients such as eggs or milk, ensure that they are stored in a cool temperature at all times.
- Do not store cottage cheese or yogurt for more than three days in the freezer.

- You can simply roast some nuts and seeds on medium flame and store them in an airtight container for snacking.

Fats

- Use healthier fats such as butter, cheese, avocado, olive oil, coconut oil, peanut butter, dark chocolate, nuts etc.
- Store them in a cool temperature.

Chapter 4: Important Steps for Meal Prep

Begin by creating a meal plan

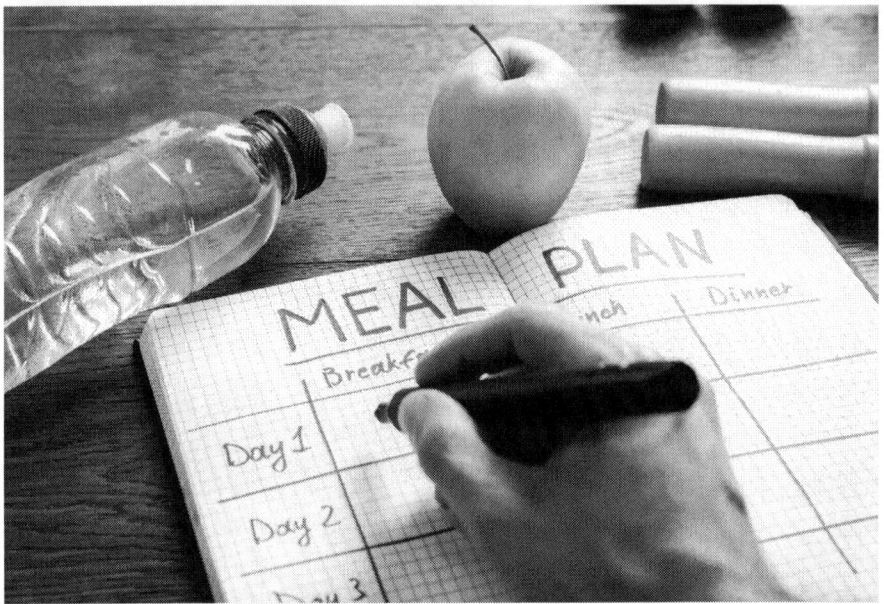

So you love the idea of meal prepping but you have never done it before? Don't worry, it's not that complicated. However, it will require you to be patient with yourself. If you are in the habit of preparing last minute meals for quite some time, you can simply reverse this habit in a day. The key is to start slowly and then gradually get hold of the meal-prepping plan. Try prepping for a day and then move on to weekly or monthly planning. Also consider the following tips while creating a plan.

- Start with a meal-planning sheet and mark the days you intend to prep your meals for.
- Have a good look at your weekly schedule. Are you attending any meeting this week? Or attending some social dos? If yes, then you may need fewer meals this week.
- For the first two weeks, just follow 2 or three breakfast recipes with similar ingredients or put together something from the leftover dinners. This will make it easier for you to adapt to your meal plan.
- Plan out some easy dinners on days you are going to be working until late.
- Prepare some snacks such as granola bars or oatmeal cookies on a weekend. You can also dry roast some nuts along with a pinch of salt and snack on it during weekdays.

Ingredients spreadsheet for grocery shopping

Okay, now we are getting a little technical about this, but trust me creating an ingredients spreadsheet is extremely beneficial. You will be thankful later. As mentioned at the beginning of the book, free download of spreadsheet template for the Weekly Meal Plan with grocery shopping list has been included as a bonus for your personal usage.

Let's have a look at a brief sample listing below. You can feel free to tweak this sheet as per your requirements.

Meat

- Chicken breasts, thighs or wings: 1 per person
- Ground beef: about 1 pound for four people
- Bacon: ½ pound for four people

Fresh produce

- Asparagus: 1 bunch
- Romaine lettuce: 1 head
- Granny Smith apple: 1
- Garlic: 2 cloves
- Onion: 1
- Avocado: half
- Lemon: Juice of one lemon
- Strawberries: One small bowl

Pantry

- Honey: ½ cup
- Canola oil: 1/8 cup
- Dijon mustard: ½ cup
- Olive oil: ¼ cup
- Italian salad dressing: 1 cup
- Balsamic vinegar: ¾ cup

- Black beans: 14 oz
- Kidney beans: 14 oz.
- Corn chips: 1 cup
- Spaghetti sauce: 1 jar
- Fresh bread: 1 loaf
- Rice: 1 cup
- Dried cranberries: 1 cup
- Diced tomatoes: 28 oz.
- Tomato paste: 8 oz.

Eggs & Dairy

- Eggs: 2 per person
- Cheddar cheese: 2 tablespoons for garnish
- Feta cheese: 4 oz.
- Butter: 4 oz.

Seasoning

- Chilli seasoning: 1 packet
- Paprika: 1 teaspoon
- Crushed red pepper: 1 teaspoon
- Rosemary: as per taste
- Salt: as per taste
- Black pepper: as per taste

Extra

- Foil: 1 sheet
- Plastic wrap: 2 sheets
- Freezer bags: as per requirement
- Plastic containers: 5 to 6

Choose your recipes wisely

Take some time out to put together your recipes. Are you planning to take up the new weight loss diet or are you going vegan? Pick recipes as per the diet you intend to follow. When you are planning your recipes, consider a few things mentioned below:

Include a cheat meal:

If you have been avoiding starchy foods or desserts for the entire week, include a cheat meal on the weekend. That's how you can reward yourself for maintaining the self-control required to stick to your diet.

Consider weather conditions:

On rainy days, hot vegetable soups can make for a perfect meal. Similarly, include some juice or coolers recipes for a hot summery afternoon.

Consider your schedule:

Don't plan on cooking complex recipes during the start of the week. Keep the meals simple and lighter during Mondays and keep the more creative ones for the weekends when you have plenty of time on your hands. The busier your schedule, the easier your recipes should be.

Kitchen space:

Choose recipes and equipment as per your kitchen space. If you have a less kitchen space, don't overcrowd it by trying to cook recipes that require a lot of chopping and pureeing. Similarly, use equipment like a hand blender instead of a food processor or iron skillet instead of huge rice cookers.

The number of recipes you chose per week should depend on the portion of food you wish to have that week. If you are cooking just for yourself, you may need fewer portions, but if you are cooking for your entire family, then you may have to double or triple the portion sizes. You can also cook different kinds of dishes using the same ingredients.

Prepare a shopping list

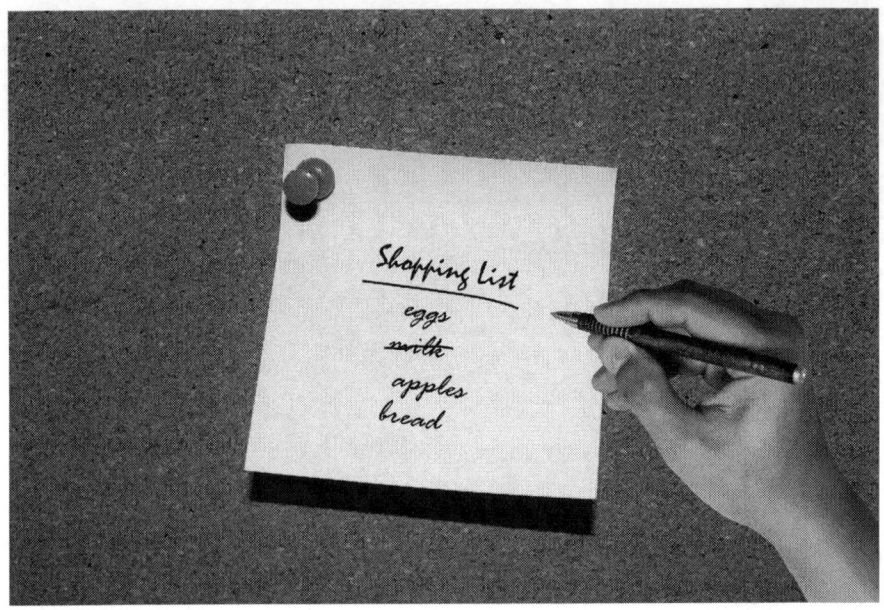

Creating a comprehensive shopping list may require some special attention. This will help you save time and energy rather than aimlessly wandering around the supermarket, trying to think of ingredients you need to buy. Moreover, you won't have to beat yourself up about the ingredients you forgot to buy after you get home. When preparing a shopping list, the first thing to consider is your budget. If you are short on cash, you can skip a few ingredients that you can do without. Condiments such as sauces, ketchup and mayonnaise can also be prepared at home with minimal ingredients, thereby saving a lot of your money. Individuals on weight loss diets will have to list down all the foods they can and cannot eat. If you buy a lot of cookies and muffins, now is the time to skip them on your shopping list. Similarly, you need more protein-rich ingredients like beef, pork or chicken. Avoid loading up on perishable foods items. Foods such as milk, cottage cheese or tofu are best not to be stored for more than three days. On the other hand, you can go generous with condiments, spices, groceries and meats.

Create an assembly line

One of the best tips for saving your cooking time is to create an assembly line. For instance, don't peel a potato, chop it and move on to the next. Instead, peel all the potatoes together, chop them all and move on to the next ingredient. Similarly, while chopping spinach or kale leaves hold them together with one hand and chop them all at once using a knife on the other hand. This method can speed up your cooking time and leave you with a lot of time in your hands. You can also use the multiple bowl method for cleaning, wherein you can use one bowl for scraps and garbage while using the other can be filled with some soap water for soaking. Lay out all the spices and condiments you are going to use on the table, so you don't have to hunt for them while cooking. It applies to spatulas, plates, dishes, knives, too etc.

Keeping prepped food fresh

Making sure that the prepped food doesn't rot may seem like a challenge to some. But storing it won't be a problem if you know all the tricks to keep the food fresh. The best way to maintain the food fresh is to use a variety of tools for storing such as silver foils, airtight containers, plastic sheets etc. For starters, you want to focus on food that can last for about 4-5 days and something your entire family can enjoy such as pork curry, chicken curry, beef stew, pilaf and soups.

- Curries can be simply stored in an airtight container and keep them in the freezer until you are ready to use them again.
- Soups can also be stored in Tupperware bowls with an airtight lid and kept in the freezer for about three days.
- You can wrap sandwiches, burgers, rolls and wraps with silver foil and refrigerate them until ready to use.
- Rice preparations such as pilaf or risotto can be stored in a plastic container or simply be added to a large vessel and keep a lid on it.
- Meats such as beef, pork, lamb, duck, etc. usually stay fresh for 3 to 5 days in refrigerator between 34 to 40 °F temperature. You can store them for up to a year in the freezer if stored in vacuum sealed bags. Without vacuum sealer, your best option for freezer storage is to remove as much air as possible in the freezer plastic sealer bags.

This will reduce freezer burns and less ice crystals to build up. Meat must be thawed only in the fridge or in cold water. When it is thawed in room temperature, it will accelerate bacteria growth and cause premature food degradation which is dangerous for health.
- Fish or poultry can be stored similarly.
- Smoothies, juices or cold beverages can be stored in mason glass jars with an airtight lid.
- For fruits and vegetables should be kept in the crisp section of fridge to prevent cross contamination with meat.
- Avoid storing the following items in the fridge:
    - Onions (whole, unpeeled)
    - Pumpkin (whole, unpeeled)
    - Water melon (whole, un-sliced)
    - Garlic (whole, unpeeled)
    - Potatoes, Sweet potatoes (whole, unpeeled)
    - Tomatoes (whole)
    - Cucumber (whole)
    - Eggplant (whole)
    - Unripe Apricots, Bananas, Kiwi, Peaches, Mangoes, Avocados
    - Honey
    - Coffee (ground or beans)
    - Cooking oil
    - Peanut butter

- Canned tuna
- Flour
- Dried spices and herbs
- UHT Milk (sealed)

Chapter 5: How to Have Fun with Meal Preps

Meal prep can play a significant role in maintaining a steady weight. Mastering your meal plans may require a bit of effort at the start, but it's all worth it in the end. Now just because you are carefully planning everything to do with your meals doesn't mean that you can't have some fun while you are at it. Here are 5 ways you can make meal preps fun.

Theme your meals

How about a themed party to make your prep fun? Arrange a fun party based on a specific theme on a relaxed weekend. You pick a certain cuisine, a specific food item and a cooking method to go with it. For instance:

- On Mondays, you could cook Chinese using chicken in barbecue style
- On Tuesdays, it could be Italian stir fry veggies
- On Wednesdays, it can be Greek style eggs cooked in a specific sauce
- On Thursdays, it can be Lamb slow cooked in Asian style
- On Fridays, it can be Mexican style cheese quesadillas

Themed parties are extremely hassle-free as your working with limited ingredients and cook using one single method. For the party, you can use different tools for servings such as skewers, sizzler plate and cast-iron trays. Place some tissues and hand wash near the sink. You can use disposable plates if you don't wish to spend time cleaning up after the meal.

Experiment with new recipes

Are you tired of cooking the same recipes over and over? Why not try something new? Get yourself a cookbook and look for innovative recipes. You can also create your recipes by tweaking them as per your taste. If you are unable to find enough time during the weekdays, try a new recipe on a relaxed Sunday afternoon. Subscribe to a Food channel and learn how you can find new ways to cook the regular recipes.

Sometimes, simply cooking the same food using a different method can make all the difference. For example, you can roast the chicken pieces before adding it to your regular chicken curry and notice how it instantly adds a different flavor to an otherwise boring dish. If your meals lack variety, you are going to get bored very soon. This will also discourage you from sticking to your diet plan. To break the monotony, you have to keep re-inventing your meals. You can also buy some exotic spices and condiments that will bring out the best flavor of the dish.

Invest in new gadgets

How about a snazzy hand blender or a compact food processor? You think you don't need new gadgets? Think again. Using limited cooking gadgets can also be responsible for bringing boredom in your cooking style. After all, you don't want to lose that Master Chef in you, do you? Here are a few cooking gadgets that are worth the investment.

Chef knife:

What's wrong with your regular knife? That it's a regular knife and it's boring. A chef knife, on the other hand, can slice food, dice it and pretty much does it all. A chef's knife is very easy to use and will get your work done in no time. The chef's knife has sharp edges, and you may get some cuts if you aren't careful.

Food processor:

The new age food processors are compact and get everything done right from chopping, slicing, dicing to shredding and making dough. You can make your pasta dough, hummus, pesto and sauces using a food processor. This equipment is easy to clean and maintain too.

Stick blender:

A stick blender is one of the most inexpensive cooking gadgets. You can get a good quality blender for as low as $30. This device is useful for churning soups, dressings, smoothies, shakes and sauces. If you come across recipes that require you to transfer the hot liquid to a blender, use a stick blender instead. You can simply blend into the liquid in the same vessel it has been cooked in.

Dutch oven:

Dutch oven is a wonder equipment, which can help you cook healthier meals. It can perfectly braise meats without having to use too much oil. It holds the temperatures well and is extremely easy to clean.

Stand mixer:

You are going to be using this equipment a lot, probably a little more than the stick blender. But this is only if you like to bake. If you don't, you can do without a stand mixer. A stand mixer can whip butter, eggs and cake batter at cruising speed. This mixer is used a lot by pastry chefs. You can use it for almost any type of icing, whipped cream, dough, bread and pretzels.

Ongoing food rotation

If you are prepping up for weekly or monthly meals, it is vital that you plan a meal rotation schedule to avoid it form going stale. Perishable items such as certain fruits, milk or tofu need to be reused in different recipes, so they don't go stale. For instance, if you like berries a lot, include strawberries in your morning breakfast for two days and then add raspberries for the next two. This way you can ensure that you are eating most of the ingredients while saving them from rotting. Do your best to fit the same on a four days rotation period. If you are using citrus fruits, make it a point to use them in pretty much all your meal schedules.

Chapter 6: Breakfast Recipes

Chocolate Peanut Butter Cups

Serving Size: 24 | Prep Time: 10 minutes | Cook Time: 25 minutes

Nutritional Info:
Calories: 155, Fat: 5 g, Protein: 4 g, Carb: 21 g

Ingredients:

4 tablespoons chia seeds mixed with ¾ cup water or 4 large eggs
2 cups cashew milk or almond milk, unsweetened
½ cup pure maple syrup or 30 drops liquid stevia
6 cup old-fashioned oats
2 scoops chocolate protein powder
6 medium to large very ripe bananas, mashed
½ cup creamy peanut butter
1 teaspoon vanilla extract
4 tablespoons cocoa powder
A large pinch salt
2 tablespoons baking powder

Directions:

1. Add milk, peanut butter, maple syrup or stevia and vanilla into a bowl and mix until well combined.
2. Add chia seed mixture or eggs and mix well.
3. Add rest of the ingredients into a bowl and add to the bowl of peanut butter mixture.
4. Pour into greased muffin tins up to ¾.

5. Bake in a preheated oven at 350° F for about 20-25 minutes or till its done.
6. Cool on a wire rack. Remove from the molds and wrap with plastic wrap. Store in an airtight container.
7. Store in the refrigerator. It can last for 5-6 days in the refrigerator.

Baked Oatmeal Cups with Raisins and Walnuts

Serving Size: 6 | Prep Time: 15 minutes | Cook Time: 30 minutes

Nutritional Info:
Calories: 154, Fat: 7 g, Protein: 4 g, Carb: 21 g

Ingredients:

1 large egg, lightly beaten
1 large banana, mashed
1 ¼ cups old-fashioned rolled oats
¾ teaspoon baking powder
6 tablespoons walnuts, chopped
½ teaspoon vanilla extract
2 teaspoons honey
½ tablespoon ground cinnamon
¾ cup almond milk, unsweetened
2 tablespoons raisins
Non-stick cooking spray

Directions:

1. Grease 6 muffin cups with nonstick cooking spray. Set aside.
2. Mix together in a bowl, banana, egg, vanilla and honey. Whisk well and set aside.
3. Add oats, baking powder and cinnamon into another bowl. Mix well.
4. Transfer the oat mixture into the bowl of banana. Mix well.
5. Add almond milk and mix into a smooth.
6. Divide the batter into the prepared muffin cups.

7. Bake in a preheated oven at 350° F for 25-30 minutes or till done and the top is golden brown.
8. Remove from the oven and cool on a wire rack. Run a knife around the edges of muffins and invert on to a plate. Wrap each in plastic wrap.
9. Place in freezer safe bags. Freeze until use.
10. To serve: Remove from the freezer the night before and place in the refrigerator to thaw.
11. Heat in a microwave and serve.

Coconut Carrot Morning Glory Muffins

Serving Size: 6 | Prep Time: 20 minutes | Cook Time: 35 minutes

Nutritional Info:
Calories: 186, Fat: 8 g, Protein: 4 g, Carb: 28 g

Ingredients:

½ cup whole-wheat flour
1 teaspoon baking powder
¼ cup old fashioned rolled oats + extra to garnish
1 teaspoon ground cinnamon
1/8 teaspoon ground allspice
½ cup applesauce, unsweetened
1 teaspoon vanilla extract
1 cup carrots, shredded
¼ cup raisins
¼ teaspoon salt
1 large egg
2 ½ tablespoons honey
2 tablespoons coconut oil, melted
¼ cup shredded coconut, unsweetened + extra to garnish

Directions:

1. Grease a muffin tin (of 6 cups capacity) with cooking spray.
2. Add all the dry ingredients into a bowl. Mix well.
3. Add all the wet ingredients (egg, honey, vanilla and apple sauce) into another bowl.
4. Add the dry ingredients into the bowl of wet ingredients.

5. Mix well until a batter that is free from lumps is formed. Add carrots, coconut and raisins. Fold gently. Divide and pour the mixture into each of the muffin cups. Spoon about a tablespoon each of oats and coconut.
6. Bake in a preheated oven at 375°F for 25-30 minutes or a toothpick when inserted in the center comes out clean.
7. Remove the tin from the oven and cool for a while. Run a knife around the edges of the cups and remove the cakes. Serve warm.
8. Wrap the unused ones with cling wrap and transfer into a freezer safe airtight container. Place in the freezer. It can store up to 3 months.
9. To serve: Remove from the freezer and thaw. Heat in a microwave and serve.

Green Muffins

Serving Size: 12 | Prep Time: 15 minutes | Cook Time: 20 minutes

Nutritional Info:
Calories: 152, Fat: 10 g, Protein: 13 g, Carb: 2 g

Ingredients:

½ cup almond milk, unsweetened
Sea salt or Himalayan pink salt to taste
Pepper powder to taste
1 cup green bell pepper
2 cups broccoli, coarsely chopped, steamed
2 cups fresh spinach, chopped
2 dozen large eggs, lightly beaten
Non-stick cooking spray

Directions:

1. Grease 2 muffin tins (of 12 cups capacity each) cups with cooking spray.
2. Add eggs, salt, pepper and milk in a large bowl. Whisk until well combined.
3. Divide the broccoli among the prepared muffin cups. Divide and add spinach over the broccoli. Finally sprinkle bell peppers.
4. Pour the egg mixture equally into the muffin cups.
5. Bake in a preheated oven at 350° F for 25-30 minutes or until the top is golden brown.
6. Remove from the oven and cool on a wire rack. Run a knife around the edges of muffins and invert on to a plate. Wrap each unused muffin with cling wrap.

7. Place in freezer safe airtight containers or bags. Close the lid or seal the bags. Freeze until use.
8. To serve: Remove from the freezer and thaw.
9. Heat in a microwave and serve.

Tofu Scramble & Breakfast Sweet Potatoes

Serving Size: 8 | Prep Time: 15 minutes | Cook Time: 30 minutes

Nutritional Info: Without the toppings
Calories: 185, Fat: 7 g, Protein: 10 g, Carb: 22 g

Ingredients:

For the sweet potatoes:
¾ pound sweet potato, peeled, chopped into ½ inch cubes
1 teaspoon chili powder
½ tablespoon olive oil
¼ teaspoon salt or to taste

For tofu scramble:
1 small red onion, finely chopped
½ block extra firm tofu, crumbled
1 cup asparagus, chopped
1 bell pepper, finely chopped
½ teaspoon ground coriander
½ teaspoon ground cumin
Pepper to taste
Salt to taste

To serve:
Cherry tomatoes
Avocado slices
Greek yogurt

Directions:

1. Add sweet potatoes into a bowl. Add oil, chili powder and salt and toss well. Transfer the potatoes to a baking sheet. Spread it all over. Do not overlap the sweet potatoes.
2. Bake in a preheated oven at 425°F for 25-30 minutes. Turn the sweet potatoes half way through baking.
3. To make scramble: Place a nonstick pan over medium heat. Add oil. When the oil is heated, add onion, asparagus and bell pepper and sauté for a few minutes until the vegetables are tender.
4. Add rest of the ingredients and sauté for a couple of minutes.
5. Divide the sweet potatoes into 4 airtight containers. Add tofu. Close the lid and store in the refrigerator until use.
6. It can be stored up to 4 days in the refrigerator.
7. To serve: Take out a container. Transfer the contents of the container into a microwave safe dish and microwave on high for a minute.
8. Alternately, add into a pan and heat thoroughly.
9. Transfer into a bowl. Place tomatoes, avocadoes on top. Spoon some yogurt on top and serve.

Potato, Asparagus & Mushroom Hash

Serving Size: 8 | Prep Time: 40 minutes | Cook Time: 40 minutes

Nutritional Info:
Calories: 239, Fat: 11 g, Protein: 5 g, Carb: 29 g

Ingredients:

2 pounds new or baby potatoes, scrubbed, rinsed, halved if large in size
2 pounds asparagus, trimmed, cut into small pieces
2 shallots, minced
1 large onion, coarsely chopped
2 cloves garlic, minced
2 tablespoons fresh sage, chopped
½ teaspoon freshly ground pepper or to taste
½ teaspoon salt or to taste
6 tablespoons extra virgin olive oil, divided
8 ounces of mushroom, sliced
1 cup roasted red peppers, chopped
Fresh chives, chopped, to garnish

Directions:

1. Steam the potatoes in your steamer equipment until just tender (do not cook too much).
2. Remove from the steamer and cool. Cut into ½ inch pieces. Transfer into an airtight container. When the potatoes are cooled completely, close the lid and refrigerate until use. It can last for 2 days.

3. Place a large skillet over medium heat. Add 2 tablespoons oil. When the oil is heated, add asparagus, garlic, shallots and mushrooms and sauté until light brown. Transfer into an airtight container. When cool, close the lid and refrigerate until use. It can last for 2 days.
4. To use: Add remaining oil to the skillet. Add onions and potatoes and cook until the potatoes are brown. Keep scraping the bottom of the skillet to remove any brown bits that are stuck.
5. Add the mushroom mixture, red pepper, sage, pepper and salt. Heat thoroughly.
6. Garnish with chives and serve.

Vegan Omelet

Serving Size: 2 | Prep Time: 10 minutes | Cook Time: 15 minutes

Nutritional Info: For 1 omelet
Calories: 232, Fat: 7.8 g, Protein: 22 g, Carb: 22 g

Ingredients:

For omelet:
10 ounces firm silken tofu, drained, pat dried
4 large cloves garlic, minced
4 tablespoons nutritional yeast
½ teaspoon paprika
Pepper to taste
Salt to taste
4 tablespoons hummus
2 teaspoons cornstarch
1 teaspoon olive oil

For the filling:
2 ½ heaping cups vegetables of your choice, chopped
2 teaspoons olive oil
Salt to taste
Pepper to taste

To serve:
2-3 tablespoons olive oil
Salsa of your choice, as required
A handful fresh herbs of your choice, chopped
½ cup vegan Parmesan cheese, shredded

Directions:

1. To make the omelet batter: Place a skillet over medium heat. Add oil. When the oil is heated, add garlic and sauté until light golden brown.
2. Remove from heat and add the garlic into a blender. Add rest of the ingredients of the omelet into the blender and blend until smooth. Add a little water if required and blend again. The batter should not be very thick. Add water a little at a time. Transfer into an airtight container and refrigerate until use.
3. To make the filling: Place the skillet back on heat. Add oil. When the oil is heated, add vegetables, salt and pepper and sauté until tender. Remove from heat and set aside in the refrigerator in an airtight container until use.
4. To use: Remove both the containers from the refrigerator 30 minutes before cooking.
5. Place a medium size ovenproof nonstick pan over medium heat. Add 1-tablespoon oil. Swirl the pan so that the oil spreads all over the skillet.
6. When the oil is heated, pour half the omelet batter into the pan. Swirl the pan so that the batter spreads or spread with the back of a spoon carefully.
7. Cook until the edges are beginning to get dry. Remove the pan from heat and place in an oven.
8. Bake in a preheated oven at 375°F for 10-15 minutes until it cooks as per your liking.
9. Remove the pan from the oven and spread half the vegetables on it. Bake for a couple of minutes. Gently slide a spatula below the omelet to loosen it. Spoon a little salsa on it. Sprinkle herbs and cheese and fold over. Slide on to a plate and serve.
10. Repeat steps 5-9 to make the other omelet.

Breakfast Burritos

Serving Size: 8 | Prep Time: 10 minutes | Cook Time: 10 minutes

Nutritional Info:
Calories: 352, Fat: 20 g, Protein: 25 g, Carb: 22 g

Ingredients:

16 large eggs
2 tablespoons extra virgin olive oil
2 red peppers, finely minced
2 tablespoons garlic, minced
1 red onion, finely minced
8 pieces thick cut bacon, cooked until crisp
8 multigrain or whole-wheat tortillas
Salt to taste
Pepper to taste
2-3 tablespoons milk

Directions:

1. Add eggs and milk in a bowl. Whisk well.
2. Place a saucepan over medium heat. Add oil. When the oil is heated, add garlic and sauté until fragrant.
3. Add onion and red pepper and sauté until onions are translucent. Pour the egg over the onions and sauté until it is cooked. Remove from heat.
4. Place the tortillas on your work area. Divide the egg mixture among the tortillas. Place a piece of bacon each tortilla. Sprinkle cheese. Wrap tightly.

5. Wrap the burrito first in wax paper and then in foil. Place in a freezer safe airtight container. Place in the freezer. It can last for 1 month.
6. To use: Unwrap the burrito and place on a microwave safe plate. Microwave for 2-3 minutes. Turn the burrito once half way through heating.
7. Remove from the microwave and cool for a minute before serving.

Spinach and Broccoli Strata

Serving Size: 16 | Prep Time: 15 minutes | Cook Time: 25 minutes

Nutritional Info:
Calories: 233, Fat: 10 g, Protein: 14 g, Carb: 22 g

Ingredients:

8 cups broccoli florets
2 medium onions, chopped
4 cups reduced fat milk
1 teaspoon sea salt or Himalayan salt
1 teaspoon pepper powder or to taste
16 slices low sodium sprouted whole grain bread, cut into 1-inch cubes
3 tablespoons olive oil
4 cloves garlic, finely chopped
4 cups raw spinach, chopped
16 large eggs, lightly beaten
½ cup feta cheese, crumbled
Non-stick cooking spray

Directions:

1. Steam the broccoli in your steamer equipment for about 2-3 minutes until just crisp as well as tender (do not cook too long).
2. Remove from the steamer and place in an ice bath to cool. Drain. Chop broccoli and set aside.
3. Place a nonstick skillet over medium heat. Add oil. When the oil is heated, add onions and sauté until translucent.
4. Add garlic and sauté until fragrant. Turn off the heat.

5. Add eggs, spinach, broccoli, milk, salt and pepper into a bowl and mix well. Add the onion mixture and whisk again.
6. Add bread into a greased, large baking dish. Pour the egg mixture over it. Press the bread cubes down that try to float.
7. Cover the dish with foil.
8. Refrigerate until use. It can last for 2 days.
9. Remove from the refrigerator 15-20 minutes before baking.
10. Bake in a preheated oven at 350°F for 15-25 minutes or until cooked.
11. Slice and serve.

Prosciutto & Asparagus Strata

Serving Size: 16 | Prep Time: 15 minutes | Cook Time: 90 minutes

Nutritional Info:
Calories: 227, Fat: 12 g, Protein: 15 g, Carb: 13 g

Ingredients:

4 slices dense multigrain bread, cut into 1-centimeter cubes
1 cup low fat milk
2 tablespoons dry mustard
1 ½ teaspoons salt or t taste
2 tablespoons extra virgin olive oil
2 cups leeks, thinly sliced, white parts only
2 pounds thin asparagus, trimmed, cut into 1 inch pieces
6 very thin slices prosciutto, torn into strips
¼ cup fresh parsley, chopped
3 tablespoons lemon zest or to taste, grated (optional)
24 large eggs
1 cup dry white wine or low-fat milk
2 teaspoons nutmeg, freshly grated
2 teaspoons freshly ground pepper or to taste
6 cups onions, halved, thinly sliced
4 cloves garlic, minced
½ cup chives or scallions, chopped
1 cup Parmigiano-Reggiano cheese, freshly grated, divided
¼ cup fresh mint, chopped
Cooking spray

Directions:

1. Add eggs into a bowl and whisk well. Add milk, wine, mustard, salt, pepper and nutmeg. Whisk well. Add bread cubes. Press the bread cubes down that try to float.
2. Cover the dish with foil.
3. Refrigerate until use.
4. Place a nonstick skillet over medium heat. Add oil. When the oil is heated, add onions and leek and sauté until onions are translucent.
5. Add garlic and sauté until fragrant.
6. Lower heat and cook until the onions are light brown in color. It may take 30-45 minutes. Stir occasionally. Add scallions and cook for a couple of minutes. Turn off the heat.
7. Meanwhile, place a skillet with enough water to cover the asparagus over medium heat. Bring to the boil. Add asparagus and cover with a lid.
8. Simmer for 2 minutes. Drain and set aside to cool. Pat the asparagus dry with a kitchen towel.
9. Grease a large baking dish with cooking spray. Transfer the onion mixture into the dish. Spread it all over the dish. Spread the asparagus over the onion mixture. Cover with foil and refrigerate until use.
10. Remove the baking dish as well as the bowl of bread an hour before baking. Remove the foil.
11. Place the prosciutto strips over the vegetable layer.
12. Add ½ cup cheese, lemon zest, parsley and mint into the bowl of eggs and stir.
13. Pour the egg mixture over the vegetables in the baking dish.
14. Sprinkle remaining cheese.
15. Bake in a preheated oven at 350°F for 35-40 minutes or until cooked.

16. Remove from the oven and wrap the dish with foil. Let it sit for 20 minutes.
17. Slice and serve.

Pumpkin Pancakes

Serving Size: 14 | Prep Time: 15 minutes | Cook Time: 10 minutes

Nutritional Info:
Calories: 201, Fat: 8 g, Protein: 7 g, Carb: 27 g

Ingredients:

3 cups white whole-wheat flour
1 teaspoon pumpkin pie spice
½ teaspoon salt
3 cups buttermilk
½ cup pecans, toasted, chopped
2 tablespoons sugar
4 teaspoons baking powder
½ teaspoon baking soda
2 large eggs
2 cups pumpkin puree
4 tablespoons canola oil
2 teaspoons vanilla extract
Cooking spray

Directions:

1. Add all the dry ingredients into an airtight container. Mix well. Close the lid and place in a cool and dry place. It can last for a month.
2. To make batter: Add rest of the ingredients in a bowl and whisk well.
3. Add the dry ingredients into the bowl of wet ingredients and mix well. Do not over mix the batter. Fold gently until mixed.

4. Cover and set aside for 15 minutes. This batter can be refrigerated for a day.
5. Place a nonstick pan or griddle over medium heat. Spray with cooking spray.
6. Do not stir the batter. Pour about ¼ cup batter on the pan. Swirl the pan slightly for the batter to spread.
7. Slowly bubbles will appear on the pancake.
8. Cook until the underside is golden brown. Flip sides and cook the other side too.
9. Repeat steps 5-8 with the remaining batter.

Chapter 7: Snack Recipes

Monkey Cookies

Serving Size: 60 | Prep Time: 10 minutes | Cook Time: 12 minutes

Nutritional Info: For 1 cookie
Calories: 47, Fat: 1.6 g, Protein: 1.5 g, Carb: 7.5 g

Ingredients:

6 medium ripe bananas, peeled, mashed
½ cup peanut butter, creamy
2/3 cup applesauce
4 cups rolled oats
½ cup cocoa powder
2 teaspoons vanilla extract

Directions:

1. Add all the ingredients into a bowl and mix well. Set aside for 20-25 minutes.
2. Take a large cookie sheet. Bake in batches.
3. Take teaspoonful of batter and drop on the cookie sheet.
4. Bake in a preheated oven at 350°F for 10-12 minutes.
5. When done, cool and transfer into freezer safe bags. Freeze until use.
6. To use: Remove from the freezer. Take out as many as necessary. Let it thaw and come to room temperature before serving.

Ham, Swiss, and Spinach Roll Ups

Serving Size: 8 | Prep Time: 5 minutes | Cook Time: 0 minutes

Nutritional Info:
Calories: 94, Fat: 5 g, Protein: 9 g, Carb: 3 g

Ingredients:

8 slices uncured deli ham
4 slices Swiss cheese, halved
8 tablespoons hummus
16 baby spinach leaves

Directions:

1. Place the ham slices on your work area. Spread about a tablespoon of hummus over it. Place half slice of cheese and spinach leaves on top. Roll tightly and place with its seam side down in an airtight container.
2. Refrigerate until use.
3. Serve later. It can store for 2 days if refrigerated.

Tri-berry Yogurt Pops

Serving Size: 16 | Prep Time: 5 minutes | Cook Time: 2 minutes

Nutritional Info:
Calories: 54, Fat: 1 g, Protein: 0 g, Carb: 6 g

Ingredients:

2 cups water
4 cups low fat Greek yogurt
1 cup strawberries, chopped
4 raspberry flavored tea bags
1 cup blueberries
4 tablespoons agave nectar

Directions:

1. Place a saucepan with water over medium heat. Bring to the boil. Remove from heat.
2. Dip the tea bags in it. Let it steep for a while. Discard the tea bags and cool completely.
3. Add rest of the ingredients into a bowl and stir. Pour tea into it. Mix well.
4. Pour into Popsicle molds or paper cups. Place in the freezer.
5. When it is semi-frozen, insert Popsicle sticks in the mold. Place it back in the freezer.
6. Freeze until use.
7. To use: Remove from the mold and serve.

Baked Parmesan Fries

Serving Size: 8 | Prep Time: 15 minutes | Cook Time: 15 minutes

Nutritional Info: 2/3 cup
Calories: 156, Fat: 5.5 g, Protein: 6 g, Carb: 20 g

Ingredients:

2 pounds Yukon gold or red potatoes, peeled, cut into fries
4 teaspoons dried Italian seasoning
½ cup Parmesan cheese, grated
Freshly and coarsely ground pepper to taste
1 teaspoon dried thyme
1 teaspoon garlic powder
4 tablespoons extra virgin olive oil
Salt to taste

Directions:

1. Grease a baking sheet with a little oil and set aside.
2. Mix together in a bowl, Parmesan, Italian seasoning, garlic powder, salt and pepper.
3. Place potatoes on the prepared baking sheet. Bake in batches if required.
4. Drizzle oil over the potatoes.
5. Sprinkle the cheese mixture on it. Toss well. Spread it in a single layer. The potatoes should not overlap.
6. Bake in a preheated oven at 425°F for 15 minutes or until tender. Transfer into a container. Cover and set-aside until use.
7. To serve: Transfer on to a baking sheet. Broil for a few minutes in an oven until crisp and serve.

Guacamole Devilled Eggs

Serving Size: 16 | Prep Time: 15 minutes | Cook Time: 10 minutes

Nutritional Info: 1 piece
Calories: 44, Fat: 3 g, Protein: 3 g, Carb: 2 g

Ingredients:

8 eggs
6 teaspoons lemon juice
Sea salt to taste
Pepper powder to taste
1 teaspoon hot pepper sauce
1 large Hass avocado, peeled, pitted, mashed
2 teaspoons red onions, finely chopped
2 tablespoons fresh cilantro, chopped
2 tablespoons tomato, finely chopped

Directions:

1. Boil the eggs in a saucepan of water. Peel the eggs. Halve the eggs lengthwise. Scoop out the yolks and place in a bowl. Place the whites on a plate.
2. Use 4 yolks and mash it. Add avocado and mix well.
3. Add rest of the ingredients to the bowl. Divide the mixture into 16 portions. Stuff this mixture into the cavity of the eggs and place in an airtight container.
4. Refrigerate until use. It can last for 2-3 days.

Easy Baked Parmesan Mushrooms

Serving Size: 8 | Prep Time: 10 minutes | Cook Time: 20 minutes

Nutritional Info:
Calories: 132, Fat: 12 g, Protein: 5 g, Carb: 4 g

Ingredients:

2 pounds button mushrooms, medium size, rinsed, quartered or halved if bigger in size
Juice of 2 lemons
Freshly ground black pepper to taste
2 teaspoons lemon zest, grated
Salt to taste
½ cup Parmesan cheese, shredded

Directions:

1. Remove the stems from the mushrooms and use for some other recipe.
2. Place the mushroom caps on a baking sheet. Add rest of the ingredients into a bowl. Mix well. Sprinkle the mixture in the cavities of the mushrooms.
3. Bake in a preheated oven at 450° F for about 20 minutes or until the cheese melts and the mushrooms are brown. Cool and transfer into an airtight container.
4. Refrigerate until use. It can last for 4-5 days.
5. To use: Remove the mushrooms from the refrigerator and transfer on a baking sheet.
6. Bake for a few minutes until thoroughly heated and serve. Alternately, in step 2, place the mushrooms in a baking dish. Cover with foil and refrigerate until use. Bake and serve immediately.

Citrus Chicken Salad Strips

Serving Size: 6 | Prep Time: 5 minutes | Cook Time: 5 minutes

Nutritional Info: 3 ounces per serving
Calories: 57, Fat: 1 g, Protein: 9 g, Carb: 4 g

Ingredients:

For the chicken strips:
¼ cup orange juice
½ tablespoon fresh ginger, peeled, minced
½ teaspoon chili powder
2 ½ cups chicken breast slices, boneless, skinless
1 tablespoon lime juice
1 teaspoon garlic, minced
½ teaspoon ground cumin

To serve:
12 cups lettuce, torn

Directions:

1. To make chicken strips: Add all the ingredients except chicken into a bowl and mix well. Add chicken and coat well. Transfer into a freezer bag. Seal the bag and place in the refrigerator for 2-3 hours.
2. Remove from the refrigerator and discard the marinade.
3. Place a nonstick pan over medium heat. Spray with cooking spray. Add chicken strips and cook until tender for 2-3 minutes on each side.
4. Remove from heat and cool completely. Transfer into freezer safe bags and label it. Freeze until use.

5. To use: Place 2 cups lettuce on each serving plate. Divide and place the strips on the lettuce and serve.

Maple Chai Roasted Chickpeas

Serving Size: 12 | Prep Time: 10 minutes | Cook Time: 40 minutes

Nutritional Info:
Calories: 148, Fat: 7 g, Protein: 6 g, Carb: 20 g

Ingredients:

4 cups canned or cooked chickpeas, drained, rinsed, dried
2 tablespoons pure maple syrup
1 teaspoon ground cinnamon
½ teaspoon ground cloves
½ teaspoon ground black pepper
½ teaspoon salt or Himalayan salt
2 tablespoons olive oil
1 teaspoon ground ginger
½ teaspoon ground cardamom

Directions:

1. Toss together all the ingredients in a bowl. Transfer onto a lined baking sheet. Spread it in a single layer. Bake in batches if required.
2. Bake in a preheated oven at 400° F for 35-40 minutes or until dry and crunchy.
3. Shake the chickpeas every 10-12 minutes. Remove from the oven and set aside to cool.
4. Transfer into an airtight container. It can last for 7-8 days.

Honey Nut Granola

Serving Size: 9 | Prep Time: 10 minutes | Cook Time: 12 minutes

Nutritional Info: 3 tablespoons
Calories: 100, Fat: 3.5 g, Protein: 3 g, Carb: 15 g

Ingredients:

¾ cup old-fashioned oats
3 tablespoons almonds, chopped
A pinch salt
2 tablespoons honey
3 tablespoons dried fruit
2 ½ tablespoons whole-wheat flour
¼ teaspoon ground cinnamon
1 tablespoon butter, unsalted, melted
¼ teaspoon vanilla extract
Cooking spray

Directions:

1. Prepare a baking sheet by lining it with parchment paper. Spray with cooking spray. Set aside.
2. Add dry ingredients into a bowl.
3. Add wet ingredients (except dried fruits) into another bowl. Pour into the bowl of dry ingredients. Mix well. Transfer on to the prepared baking sheet. Spread it all over the baking sheet.
4. Bake in a preheated oven at 400° F for 10-12 minutes or until light brown.
5. Remove from oven and cool. Break into pieces and mix dried fruit.
6. Transfer into an airtight container until use.

Parmesan Carrot Fries

Serving Size: 8 | Prep Time: 15 minutes | Cook Time: 15 minutes

Nutritional Info:
Calories: 83, Fat: 3 g, Protein: 2 g, Carb: 11 g

Ingredients:

2 pounds carrots, peeled, cut into thin fries
Freshly cracked pepper to taste
3 tablespoons olive oil
Coarse sea salt to taste
6 tablespoons Parmesan cheese, freshly grated
¼ cup fresh basil leaves, chopped

Directions:

1. Grease a baking sheet with a little oil and set aside.
2. Mix together in a bowl, carrots, oil, salt and pepper.
3. Place carrots on the prepared baking sheet. Bake in batches if required.
4. Bake in a preheated oven at 400°F for 12-15 minutes or until tender. Transfer into a container. Cover and set-aside until use.
5. To serve: Heat for a few minutes in an oven.
6. Sprinkle basil and Parmesan cheese and serve.

Asian Turkey Lettuce Wraps

Serving Size: 12 | Prep Time: 10 minutes | Cook Time: 15 minutes

Nutritional Info:
Calories: 171, Fat: 9 g, Protein: 15 g, Carb: 9 g

Ingredients:

Iceberg lettuce leaves, as required
2 pounds ground turkey
2 tablespoons onion powder
½ cup hoisin sauce
2 tablespoons rice wine vinegar
4 teaspoons dark sesame oil
Sriracha sauce to taste
2 tablespoons olive oil
1 teaspoon garlic powder
2 tablespoons soy sauce
2 teaspoons ginger, grated
2 bunches green onions, thinly sliced
1 large carrot, peeled, shredded

Directions:

1. Place a skillet over medium high heat. Add olive oil. When the oil is heated, add turkey and cook until brown.
2. Add onion powder, garlic powder, ginger, sesame oil, vinegar, hoisin sauce and soy sauce. Sauté for a few minutes.
3. Add sriracha sauce and green onions. Sauté until the green onion wilts.
4. Cool completely and transfer into an airtight container. Refrigerate until use. It can last for 3 days. You can also freeze it for a longer timer.

5. To use: Remove the turkey mixture from the refrigerator an hour before serving. Thaw completely if frozen.
6. Place lettuce cups on your work area.
7. Spoon some of the turkey mixture and place some carrots.
8. Place in a baking dish and microwave for a few seconds to heat.
9. Serve.

Healthy Cookie Dough Peanut Butter Protein Balls

Serving Size: 24 | Prep Time: 5 minutes | Cook Time: 0 minutes

Nutritional Info: 1 ball
Calories: 135, Fat: 9.2 g, Protein: 5.5 g, Carb: 5.9 g

Ingredients:

1 ½ cups all-natural drippy peanut butter or any other type nut butter of your choice
1 cup protein powder
2 tablespoons unsweetened almond milk + extra if required
2 tablespoons coconut flour + extra if required
2 teaspoons vanilla extract
¼ cup chocolate chips

Directions:

1. Add all the ingredients except chocolate chips into a bowl and mix well.
2. Add a little more milk if the mixture is very dry or add a little more coconut flour if the mixture is very wet. You should be able to form balls. Add accordingly to your choice.
3. Add chocolate chips and mix well.
4. Divide the mixture into 24 equal portions. Shape each portion into a ball and place in an airtight container.
5. Refrigerate until use.

Sweet Potato Hummus

Serving Size: 12 | Prep Time: 5 minutes | Cook Time: 0 minutes

Nutritional Info: Only for hummus
Calories: 212, Fat: 13 g, Protein: 5 g, Carb: 21 g

Ingredients:

3 cups cooked garbanzo beans
4 tablespoons tahini
4 tablespoons sriracha sauce
¼ teaspoon paprika
¼ cup fresh thyme, chopped
1 cup sweet potato puree
4 tablespoons extra virgin olive oil
¼ teaspoon salt or to taste
1 teaspoon garlic powder
6 tablespoons fresh goat's cheese

Directions:

1. Add garbanzo beans, sweet potato puree, tahini, olive oil and sriracha sauce into a blender and blend until smooth. Scrape the sides of the blender with a spatula.
2. Add some more olive oil if the mixture is too thick. Add a little at a time and blend each time.
3. Add garlic powder, thyme and paprika and blend again.
4. Transfer into a bowl. Sprinkle goat's cheese on top.
5. Cover and refrigerate until use. It can last for 3-5 days.
6. To serve: Serve with crackers or vegetable sticks.

White Bean and Roasted Red Pepper Hummus

Serving Size: 14 | Prep Time: 5 minutes | Cook Time: 0 minutes

Nutritional Info: Only for hummus
Calories: 96, Fat: 5 g, Protein: 3 g, Carb: 11 g

Ingredients:

2 cans (15 ounces each) white beans or cannellini beans, drained, rinsed
4 teaspoons fresh rosemary, finely chopped
1 jar (12 ounces) roasted red peppers packed in water, drained
4 tablespoons olive oil
8 cloves garlic, coarsely chopped

Directions:

1. Add beans, rosemary, peppers and garlic into a blender and blend until smooth.
2. With the blender running, pour oil in a thin stream. Blend until smooth.
3. Transfer into a bowl.
4. Cover and refrigerate until use. It can last for 3-5 days.
5. To serve: Serve with fresh vegetable sticks like carrots, cucumber etc.

Mini Peanut Butter and Apple Sandwich

Serving Size: 8 | Prep Time: 5 minutes | Cook Time: 20 minutes

Nutritional Info: For 2 sandwiches
Calories: 200, Fat: 8 g, Protein: 5 g, Carb: 32 g

Ingredients:

½ cup old fashioned rolled oats
½ teaspoon ground cinnamon
1 tablespoon orange juice
½ tablespoon packed brown sugar
¼ teaspoon vanilla extract
2 tablespoons raisins
½ teaspoon lemon juice (optional)
1 tablespoon ground flaxseeds
A pinch sea salt
1 tablespoon honey
½ teaspoon vegetable oil
2 medium apples
3 tablespoons creamy peanut butter
2 medium apples, cored, cut each apple into 8 slices of ¼ inch thick, to serve
Cooking spray

Directions:

1. Add oats, ground flaxseeds, cinnamon and salt into a bowl.
2. Add honey, orange juice, and brown sugar into a small saucepan. Place the saucepan over medium heat. Heat until the sugar dissolves completely. Stir simultaneously.
3. Turn off the heat. Add vanilla and oil and stir.

4. Pour this mixture over the oats mixture. Mix until well coated.
5. Transfer on to a greased baking sheet.
6. Bake in a preheated oven at 300°F for 20 minutes or until golden brown. Transfer into an airtight container. Set aside in a cool dark place at room temperature until use. It can last for 2 weeks.
7. To serve: Brush apple slices with lemon juice. Spread peanut butter on half the slices of apple.
8. Sprinkle granola on it. Cover with the remaining apple slices and press lightly.
9. Serve.

Broccoli Parmesan Meatballs

Serving Size: 24 | Prep Time: 20 minutes | Cook Time: 20 minutes

Nutritional Info: For 1 meatball
Calories: 64, Fat: 4.4 g, Protein: 4.8 g, Carb: 2.4 g

Ingredients:

1 cup raw almonds
1 cup Parmesan cheese, shredded
Salt to taste
Pepper to taste
Cooking spray or olive oil to grease
4 cups broccoli florets, steamed
4 cloves garlic, minced
2 eggs, lightly beaten

Directions:

1. Add almonds into the food processor and pulse until coarse. Transfer into a bowl.
2. Add broccoli into the food processor and pulse until finely chopped. Transfer into the bowl of almonds. Add rest of the ingredients and mix well.
3. Grease 2 mini muffin tins (of 12 muffins capacity) with oil or cooking spray.
4. Divide the mixture and form 24 balls. Place in the muffin tins.
5. Bake in a preheated oven at 350°F for 20 minutes or until golden brown. Remove from the oven and cool for a few minutes. Run a knife around the edges of the muffins to loosen them. Cool completely.

6. Transfer into an airtight container. Refrigerate until use. It can last for 2-3 days.
7. To use: Heat in the microwave and serve.

Chapter 8: Lunch Recipes

Chicken and Black Bean Burrito Salad in a Mason jar

Serving Size: 8 | Prep Time: 20 minutes | Cook Time: 20 minutes

Nutritional Info:
Calories: 273, Fat: 8 g, Protein: 20 g, Carb: 33 g

Ingredients:

For salad:
4 cups canned black beans
2 cups jicama, chopped
2 cups red onions, thinly sliced
16 cups romaine lettuce, chopped or torn
8 ounces chicken breasts, cooked, shredded
1 cup radish, thinly sliced
2 cups cherry tomatoes, halved
½ cup cheddar cheese, shredded

For dressing:
1 cup fresh lemon juice
2 cloves garlic, chopped
2 tablespoons extra virgin olive oil
1 ¼ cups fresh cilantro, chopped, divided
2 medium jalapenos, deseeded, chopped

Directions:

1. To make dressing: Set aside 1 cup of cilantro and add ¼ cup cilantro along with garlic and jalapenos into the blender and blend until smooth.
2. With the blender running, slowly pour the oil in a thin stream. Blend until well combined.
3. Take 8 mason's jars and divide the dressing among the jars.
4. Layer all the salad ingredients in any manner you desire. Top with the remaining cilantro. Do not stir. Fasten the lids on the jars.
5. Refrigerate until use. It lasts for 3 days.
6. To use: Stir and serve.

BLT Pasta Salad

Serving Size: 4 | Prep Time: 10 minutes | Cook Time: 15 minutes

Nutritional Info:
Calories: 323, Fat: 13 g, Protein: 18 g, Carb: 35 g

Ingredients:

3½ ounces bow tie pasta
1½ ounces spinach
2 tablespoons crème fraiche
8 bacon rashers, cooked until crisp, broken or chopped
24 cherry tomatoes, halved
2 teaspoons whole grain mustard
Salt to taste

Directions:

1. Cook pasta according to the instructions on the package.
2. Add all the ingredients into a bowl and mix well.
3. Transfer into an airtight container and refrigerate until use. It can last for 2 days.

Greek Courgetti Salad

Serving Size: 4 | Prep Time: 5 minutes | Cook Time: 0 minutes

Nutritional Info:
Calories: 293, Fat: 25 g, Protein: 6 g, Carb: 5 g

Ingredients:

1 cucumber, sliced diagonally
14 ounces marinated olives with sun dried tomatoes
4¼ ounces feta cheese, crumbled
17½ ounces courgette (noodles made from courgette)
Seasoning of your choice
Extra virgin olive oil to drizzle

Directions:

1. Layer the ingredients in 4 mason's jars in whatever manner you desire. Drizzle oil on top.
2. Fasten the lid and refrigerate until use. It can last for 2 days.
3. Stir and serve.

Griddled Salad Jar

Serving Size: 8 | Prep Time: 10 minutes | Cook Time: 5 minutes

Nutritional Info:
Calories: 292, Fat: 23 g, Protein: 8 g, Carb: 11 g

Ingredients:

For salad:
1 medium eggplant, sliced
1 tomato, chopped
½ courgette, sliced
½ tablespoon olive oil
3½ ounces feta cheese, crumbled
1¾ ounces kalamata olives
4½ ounces canned or cooked chickpeas
1 small cucumber, deseeded, chopped
A handful of mint leaves, torn or chopped
1 small yellow bell pepper, deseeded, chopped
¾ ounce sundried tomatoes
A handful of dill leaves, chopped
Salt to taste
Pepper to taste

For pickled onion dressing:
½ red onion, thinly sliced
2 tablespoons white wine vinegar
3½ tablespoons extra virgin olive oil
¼ teaspoon coriander seeds
2 tablespoons lemon juice

Directions:

1. To make pickled onion dressing: Add all the ingredients of the dressing into a small pan. Place the pan over medium low heat. Heat until the onions are translucent and slightly soft.
2. Turn off heat and set aside.
3. Brush eggplant and courgette slices with olive oil.
4. Place a griddle pan over medium high heat. When the pan begins to smoke, place eggplant and courgette slices on it.
5. Cook on both the sides until slightly charred. Remove on to a plate. Sprinkle salt and pepper and set aside.
6. Add lemon juice and onion into the cooled onion mixture. Add salt and pepper and stir.
7. Divide into 8 mason's jars.
8. Divide and place tomatoes, feta, chickpeas and olives in the jars. Press slightly with a spoon to push the salad.
9. Spoon some sundried tomatoes along with a little of its oil. Next layer with the griddled vegetables. Next place cucumber, followed by bell pepper and finally mint and dill leaves.
10. Fasten the lid and refrigerate until use. It can last for 2 days.
11. To serve: Empty the jars into individual serving bowls. Toss well and serve.

Creamy Radish Soup

Serving Size: 8 | Prep Time: 10 minutes | Cook Time: 25 minutes

Nutritional Info:
Calories: 230, Fat: 10 g, Protein: 6 g, Carb: 22 g

Ingredients:

4 cups radish, sliced, divided
16 ounces Yukon gold potatoes, peeled, chopped into 1-inch cubes
1 cup onions, chopped
4 tablespoons extra virgin olive oil
½ cup low fat sour cream
Salt to taste
White or black pepper to taste
4 cups low fat milk
2 tablespoons fresh radish greens, chopped to serve

Directions:

1. Cut about ½ cup of radish into matchsticks and place in a small airtight container. Refrigerate until use. Chop the remaining radishes.
2. Place a large saucepan over medium high heat. Add oil. When the oil is heated, add 3 ½ cups radish and onion and sauté until the onions are brown and radish are slightly tender.
3. Add potatoes, salt, pepper and milk and stir. Bring to the boil. Stir a couple of times while it is boiling.
4. Lower heat and cover with a lid. Cook until the potatoes are tender. Turn off the heat.
5. Cool slightly. Blend the contents with an immersion blender until smooth. Alternately, transfer into a blender and blend until smooth.

6. Heat the soup thoroughly. Remove from heat. Cool completely. Transfer into a container and refrigerate until use. It can last for 2 days.
7. To use: Heat thoroughly. Ladle into soup bowls. Place some of the matchstick radish (that was set aside) in each bowl.
8. Drizzle about a tablespoon of sour cream in each bowl. Sprinkle radish greens on top and serve.

Carrot and Ginger Immune Boosting Soup

Serving Size: 4 | Prep Time: 5 minutes | Cook Time: 5 minutes

Nutritional Info:
Calories: 223, Fat: 7 g, Protein: 5 g, Carb: 30 g

Ingredients:

12 large carrots, peeled, chopped
1 ½ teaspoons turmeric powder
3 ounces whole meal bread, chopped
3 cups vegetable stock
4 tablespoons ginger, peeled, grated
1/8 teaspoon cayenne pepper + extra to garnish
4 tablespoons sour cream + extra to garnish

Directions:

1. Place carrots, ginger and whole meal bread in different airtight containers in the refrigerator. It can last for 3-4 days. Place sour cream and stock in the refrigerator.
2. Keep rest of the ingredients on hand.
3. To use: Add all the ingredients including the refrigerated ingredients into a blender and blend until smooth.
4. Pour into a saucepan and place the saucepan over medium heat.
5. Heat thoroughly.
6. Ladle into soup bowls. Drizzle sour cream and sprinkle cayenne pepper and serve.

Green Soup with Chicken

Serving Size: 10 | Prep Time: 15 minutes | Cook Time: 30 minutes

Nutritional Info:
Calories: 226, Fat: 9 g, Protein: 19 g, Carb: 18 g

Ingredients:

3 tablespoons extra virgin olive oil, divided
2 large cloves garlic, chopped
1 large carrot, chopped
1 medium red bell pepper, chopped
2 large chicken breasts, skinless, quartered
10 cups low sodium chicken broth
3 teaspoons dried marjoram
2 cans (15 ounces each) canned cannellini beans or great northern beans, rinsed
12 ounces baby spinach, chopped
2/3 cup fresh basil leaves, chopped
½ cup Parmesan, grated
Freshly ground pepper to taste
Salt to taste
Multigrain croutons to serve (optional)

Directions:

1. Place a large saucepan over medium high heat. Add half the oil. When the oil is heated, add carrot, bell pepper and chicken and sauté until the chicken is brown. Add garlic and sauté for about a minute until fragrant.
2. Add broth and marjoram and bring to the boil.
3. Lower heat and cover with a lid. Simmer until chicken is cooked. Remove the chicken with a slotted spoon and place on your work area. When cool enough to handle, shred with a pair of forks.

4. Meanwhile, add spinach and beans into the saucepan and cook until the spinach wilts. Add chicken and pepper. Heat thoroughly. Cool and refrigerate until use. Can last for 3-4 days if refrigerated and 2-3 months if frozen.
5. To make pesto: Add remaining oil into the blender. Add Parmesan and basil and pulse until you get a coarse texture. Add a little water and pulse again. Transfer into an airtight container and refrigerate until use. It can last for 3 days.
6. To use: Remove the soup and pesto from the refrigerator. Thaw if frozen. Heat the soup thoroughly.
7. Ladle into individual soup bowls. Drizzle pesto and swirl with a spoon.
8. Top with croutons and serve.

Turkey and Spring Onion Wraps

Serving Size: 8 | Prep Time: 10 minutes | Cook Time: 1 minutes

Nutritional Info:
Calories: 267, Fat: 9 g, Protein: 24 g, Carb: 25 g

Ingredients:

4 tablespoons low fat mayonnaise
8 curly lettuce leaves
12 spring onions, thinly sliced
8 flour tortillas
4 tablespoons pesto – refer above recipe for pesto or use store bought ones
17½ ounces cooked turkey, shredded
2 medium cucumbers, peeled, shredded

Directions:

1. Add mayonnaise and pesto into a bowl and mix well. Set aside
2. Spread the tortillas on your work area. Divide rest of the ingredients and place on the tortillas. Spoon the mayonnaise mixture on it.
3. Roll and place in an airtight container with its seam side down.
4. Refrigerate until use. It can last for 2 days.
5. To use: Microwave for a few seconds and serve.

Carrot and Hummus Roll Ups

Serving Size: 8 | Prep Time: 15 minutes | Cook Time: 1 minutes

Nutritional Info:
Calories: 355, Fat: 19 g, Protein: 10 g, Carb: 37 g

Ingredients:

14 ounces hummus
8 carrots, grated
8 seeded wraps
1 bunch rocket lettuce, torn
Seasoning of your choice

Directions:

1. Place the wraps on your work area. Spread hummus over it. Sprinkle carrots and lettuce leaves.
2. Sprinkle seasoning on it. Roll tightly and place in an airtight container.
3. Refrigerate until use. It can last for 2 days.
4. To use: Microwave for a few seconds and serve.

Prawn Sweet Chili Noodle Salad

Serving Size: 3 | Prep Time: 10 minutes | Cook Time: 5 minutes

Nutritional Info:
Calories: 267, Fat: 5 g, Protein: 20 g, Carb: 39 g

Ingredients:

1 ½ nests medium egg noodles
½ bunch spring onions, thinly sliced
1¾ ounces cherry tomatoes, halved
7 ounces king prawns, cooked, thaw if frozen
2 tablespoons sweet chili sauce
2 tablespoons cashews, roasted, broken into pieces
1 small cucumber, halved lengthwise, deseeded, cut into half moons
Zest of a lime, grated
Juice of a lime
1 green chili, deseeded, finely chopped
3½ ounces baby spinach leaves, rinsed

Directions:

1. Cook the noodles according to the instructions on the package for 4 minutes. Drain and rinse under cold water. Drain and set aside in a bowl. Chop into smaller pieces with a scissors if you desire.
2. Add cucumber, onions, chili, tomatoes and prawn into the bowl of noodles and toss.
3. Mix together in a small bowl, lime juice, lime zest and chili sauce. Pour over the noodles and fold gently.
4. Refrigerate until use. It can last for a day.

5. To serve: Divide the spinach among individual serving plates. Place noodles and sprinkle cashews on top and serve.

Vegetarian Reuben with Russian dressing

Serving Size: 4 | Prep Time: 20 minutes | Cook Time: 10 minutes

Nutritional Info: For 1 sandwich
Calories: 343, Fat: 12 g, Protein: 16 g, Carb: 44 g

Ingredients:

For Russian dressing:
4 tablespoons low fat mayonnaise
4 teaspoons capers, chopped
4 teaspoons ketchup
2 teaspoons chopped pickle or relish

For sandwiches:
6 teaspoons extra virgin olive oil, divided
2 cups mushrooms, sliced
Freshly ground pepper to taste
1 cup low fat Swiss cheese, shredded
2 small red onions, thinly sliced
10 cups baby spinach
8 slices rye bread
1 cup sauerkraut

Directions:

1. To make Russian dressing: Add mayonnaise and ketchup into a bowl and whisk until well combined. Add capers and pickle and mix well. Transfer into an airtight container and refrigerate until use. It can last for 2 days.

2. Have rest of the ingredients on hand. Place spinach, sauerkraut, cheese and mushrooms in different airtight containers in the refrigerator until use.
3. To use: Place a large nonstick skillet over medium high heat. Add 4 teaspoons oil. When the oil is heated, add onions and mushrooms and sauté until tender. Add spinach and cook until spinach wilts.
4. Transfer on to a plate.
5. Place the pan back on heat. Add remaining oil. When the oil is heated, place bread slices in the pan. Divide and place the cheese slices over the bread.
6. Divide and spread sauerkraut on 4 bread slices. Divide and spread spinach mixture on the remaining 4 slices of bread. Cook until the cheese melts and the underside is golden brown.
7. Add the dressing on the bread slices with spinach. Place the bread slices with sauerkraut over the bread slices with spinach. Cut into 2 halves or triangles.
8. Serve.

Sesame Noodles

Serving Size: 4 | Prep Time: 20 minutes | Cook Time: 20 minutes

Nutritional Info:
Calories: 340, Fat: 12 g, Protein: 12 g, Carb: 50 g

Ingredients:

½ pound whole-wheat spaghetti
1 tablespoons sesame oil
1 tablespoon rice wine vinegar or lime juice
½ bunch scallions, sliced, divided
2 cups snow peas, trimmed, sliced on the bias
¼ cup sesame seeds, toasted
¼ cup low sodium soy sauce
1 tablespoon canola oil
¾ teaspoon crushed red pepper or to taste
A handful of fresh cilantro, chopped
1 small red bell pepper, thinly sliced

Directions:

1. Cook spaghetti according to the instructions on the package until al dente. Drain and rinse in cold water. Drain again and set aside in the refrigerator until use.
2. Have the Snowpeas and bell peppers ready and refrigerate until use.
3. Add soy sauce, canola oil, sesame oil, crushed red pepper and vinegar into a bowl. Whisk well. Add a little of the scallions and a little cilantro and stir. Refrigerate until use. Use all the refrigerated ingredients within a day.

4. To use: Remove all the ingredients from the refrigerator at least an hour before mixing.
5. Add all the refrigerated ingredients into a bowl and toss well. Add sesame seeds and toss again. Sprinkle remaining scallions and some cilantro on top and serve.

Maple Roasted Sweet Potatoes

Serving Size: 3 | Prep Time: 10 minutes | Cook Time: 70 minutes

Nutritional Info: ½ cup
Calories: 92, Fat: 2 g, Protein: 1 g, Carb: 18 g

Ingredients:

1 ¼ pounds sweet potatoes, peeled, cut into 1 ½ inch pieces
1 tablespoon butter, melted
¼ teaspoon salt or to taste
2½ tablespoons maple syrup
½ tablespoon lemon juice
Freshly ground pepper to taste

Directions:

1. Spread the sweet potato pieces in a glass baking dish.
2. Mix together rest of the ingredients in a bowl and pour over the sweet potatoes. Mix until the sweet potatoes are well coated with the mixture. Cover with foil.
3. Bake in a preheated oven 400° F for about 12 minutes. Uncover and bake for another 40-50 minutes. Turn the sweet potatoes every 10-15 minutes. It should be tender inside and brown outside.
4. When done, remove from the oven. Cool completely. Transfer into an airtight container. Refrigerate until use. It can last for a day.
5. To serve: Broil in a preheated oven for a few minutes until crisp on the outside. Turn the sweet potatoes after a few minutes.

Easy Pasta Salad

Serving Size: 8 | Prep Time: 10 minutes | Cook Time: 12 minutes

Nutritional Info:
Calories: 292, Fat: 7 g, Protein: 10 g, Carb: 51 g

Ingredients:

2 pounds pasta
2 bunches parsley, chopped
Juice of 2 lemons
Zest of 2 lemons, grated
¾ pound frozen green peas
1 medium packet chives, snipped
4 tablespoons olive oil
Seasoning of your choice, as required

Directions:

1. Cook pasta according to the instructions on the package. Add peas during the last 2 minutes of cooking. Drain and rinse in cold water. Drain and transfer into a bowl.
2. Add rest of the ingredients and toss well. Transfer into an airtight container.
3. Refrigerate until use. It can last for 3-4 days.
4. To use: Serve at either room temperature or chilled.

Chapter 9: Dinner Recipes

Miso Noodle Soup

Serving Size: 4 | Prep Time: 4 minutes | Cook Time: 2 minutes

Nutritional Info:
Calories: 223, Fat: 7.7 g, Protein: 9 g, Carb: 32 g

Ingredients:

4 tablespoons white miso mixed with 2 tablespoons warm water
4 teaspoons sesame oil, toasted
1 1/3 cup red cabbage, thinly sliced
8 shiitake mushroom caps, thinly sliced
16 thin slices jalapeño
2 large hardboiled egg, chopped
2 cloves garlic, grated
2 cups cooked flat brown rice (or 4 ounces uncooked pad Thai noodles)
2 green onions, thinly sliced
2 tablespoons fresh cilantro, chopped
Boiling hot water to serve

Directions:

1. Mix together oil, miso and garlic in a bowl and divide among 4 wide jars of 1 pint each.
2. Layer with the remaining ingredients in any manner you desire.
3. Close the lid tightly and place in the refrigerator until use. It can last for 2-3 days.

4. To serve: Pour boiling hot water into the jars. Do not fill right up to the top. Leave about an inch from the top. Cover with lid and let it sit for 2 minutes before serving.

Chickpea and Sausage Pesto Soup

Serving Size: 2 | Prep Time: 10 minutes | Cook Time: 2 minutes

Nutritional Info:
Calories: 390, Fat: 20.1 g, Protein: 20 g, Carb: 33 g

Ingredients:

1 cup canned or cooked chickpeas, rinsed, drained
4 tablespoons refrigerated prepared pesto – refer Green chicken soup recipe
2/3 cup Swiss chard, thinly sliced
½ cup carrots cut into matchsticks
4 ounces cooked sundried tomato chicken sausage, diced
6 grape tomatoes, quartered
Boiling hot water to serve

Directions:

1. Divide all the ingredients between 2 wide jars of 1 pint each.
2. Layer the ingredients in any manner you desire.
3. Close the lid tightly and place in the refrigerator until use. It can last for 2-3 days.
4. To serve: Pour boiling hot water into the jars. Do not fill right up to the top. Leave about an inch from the top. Cover with lid and let it sit for 2 minutes before serving.

Split Pea Soup

Serving Size: 12 | Prep Time: 10 minutes | Cook Time: 75 minutes

Nutritional Info:
Calories: 277.8, Fat: 3.9 g, Protein: 27 g, Carb: 33.7 g

Ingredients:

3 cups green or yellow split peas, rinsed, soaked in water overnight, drained
2 pounds extra lean ground turkey
2 large carrots, diced
2 large onions, minced
2 bay leaves
12 cups water
2 teaspoons liquid smoke
Freshly ground black pepper to taste
Salt to taste
Cooking spray

Directions:

1. Add split peas into a large pot or Dutch oven. Place the pot over medium heat. Add water and bay leaves and bring to the boil.
2. Lower heat and cover with a lid.
3. Simmer until the split peas are tender. It will take approximately 45 minutes.
4. Meanwhile, place a skillet over medium heat. Spray with cooking spray. Add onions and sauté until soft. Remove the onions and place in a bowl. Set aside.
5. Place the skillet back over heat. Add turkey and sauté until golden brown. Break it simultaneously as it cooks.
6. Add the onions that were set aside, carrots, salt, pepper and liquid smoke. Transfer into the soup pot. Stir well.

7. Cover and cook until the carrots are tender. Discard the bay leaves. Cool completely and transfer into an airtight container. It can last for 4 days if refrigerated and 3 months if frozen.
8. Heat thoroughly before use. Ladle into individual soup bowls. Serve with sprouted, toasted bread.

Vegan Chili

Serving Size: 10 | Prep Time: 10 minutes | Cook Time: 20 minutes

Nutritional Info:
Calories: 171, Fat: 0 g, Protein: 20 g, Carb: 23 g

Ingredients:

1 pound seitan
1 small onion, chopped
1 habanero chili, deseeded, deveined, chopped
¼ teaspoon paprika
Pepper powder to taste
½ teaspoon chili powder
2 cloves garlic, finely chopped
½ teaspoon salt or to taste
7½ ounces canned kidney beans with its liquid
7½ ounces canned black beans with its liquid
1 medium tomato, chopped
Non-stick cooking spray

Directions:

1. Add seitan into the food processor bowl and process until you get a texture that is like ground beef. Transfer into a bowl and set aside.
2. Place a skillet over medium high heat. Spray with cooking spray.
3. Add onions and sauté until pink. Add garlic, ground seitan and habanero and sauté until seitan is golden brown.
4. Add rest of the ingredients and simmer until heated thoroughly.

5. Remove from heat and cool completely. Transfer into freezer safe zip lock bags and seal the bags. Freeze until use.
6. To serve: Remove the bags from the freezer and thaw for a while. Empty the contents into a saucepan. Heat thoroughly and serve.

Sweet Potato Casserole

Serving Size: 5 | Prep Time: 15 minutes | Cook Time: 80 minutes

Nutritional Info:
Calories: 238, Fat: 9 g, Protein: 5 g, Carb: 36 g

Ingredients:

1 ¼ pounds sweet potatoes, peeled cut into 2-inch chunks
½ tablespoon canola oil
¼ cup low fat milk
½ teaspoon vanilla extract
¼ cup whole-wheat flour
2 teaspoons orange juice concentrate
½ tablespoon butter, melted
1 large egg
½ tablespoon honey
1 teaspoon orange zest, freshly grated
¼ teaspoon salt
2½ tablespoons packed brown sugar
¼ cup pecans, chopped
Cooking spray

Directions:

1. Place a saucepan over medium heat. Add sweet potatoes and fill with water. Bring to the boil.
2. Cover and cook until soft. Drain and add it back into the pot. Mash the sweet potatoes with a potato masher.
3. Grease a baking dish with cooking spray. Set aside.

4. Add egg, honey and oil into a bowl and whisk well. Add sweet potatoes and mix well. Add milk, vanilla, zest and salt and mix. Transfer into the prepared baking dish. Spread it all over the dish.
5. To make topping: Add rest of the ingredients into a small bowl. Mix well with your fingers until the mixture is crumbly in texture. Sprinkle over the sweet potato layer in the dish.
6. Cover and refrigerate until use.
7. To use: Bake in a preheated oven 450° F for about 20 minutes or until golden brown in color.

Classic Dinner Pancakes

Serving Size: 12 | Prep Time: 5 minutes | Cook Time: 5 minutes

Nutritional Info:
Calories: 230, Fat: 8.8 g, Protein: 8.2 g, Carb: 29.2 g

Ingredients:

For dry ingredients:
3 cups whole wheat pastry flour or flour
1 ½ teaspoons salt
2 teaspoons baking soda
2 tablespoons sugar

For wet ingredients:
6 eggs
3 1/3 cups buttermilk
6 tablespoons butter, melted

Directions:

1. Add all the dry ingredients into an airtight container. Mix well. Close the lid and place in a cool and dry place until use. It can last for a month.
2. To make batter: Add all the wet ingredients into a bowl and whisk well.
3. Add the dry ingredients into the bowl of wet ingredients and mix well. Do not over mix the batter. Fold gently until mixed.
4. Cover and set aside for 15 minutes. This batter can be refrigerated for a day.

5. Place a nonstick pan or griddle over medium heat. Spray with cooking spray.
6. Do not stir the batter. Pour about ¼ cup batter on the pan. Swirl the pan slightly for the batter to spread.
7. Slowly bubbles will appear on the pancake.
8. Cook until the underside is golden brown. Flip sides and cook the other side too.
9. Repeat steps 5-8 with the remaining batter.
10. Serve pancakes with any curry or with maple syrup.

Note: Nutritional value of curry or maple syrup not included.

Potato Rounds with Fresh Lemon

Serving Size: 8 | Prep Time: 15 minutes | Cook Time: 20 minutes

Nutritional Info:
Calories: 130, Fat: 3.5 g, Protein: 3 g, Carb: 21 g

Ingredients:

2 pounds fingerling potatoes, scrubbed, sliced into 1/8 inch thick rounds

4 teaspoons dried oregano

4 teaspoons lemon zest, grated

2 tablespoons extra virgin olive oil, divided

Coarsely ground black pepper to taste

Salt to taste

Directions:

1. Line a baking sheet with foil.
2. Add potatoes into a bowl. Pour half the oil on it and toss well. Season with pepper and oregano and toss well.
3. Transfer on to the prepared baking sheet. Spread it in a single layer. Bake in batches if required.
4. Bake in a preheated oven 450° F for about 20 minutes or until golden brown in color. It should be tender inside and crisp outside. Turn the potatoes half way through baking.
5. When done, remove from the oven. Transfer into an airtight container. Refrigerate until use. It can last for 4-5 days.
6. To serve: Broil in a preheated oven for a few minutes until crisp on the outside. Turn the potatoes after a few minutes.
7. Sprinkle remaining oil, lemon zest and salt and toss well. Serve immediately.

Baked Mac & Cheese

Serving Size: 8 | Prep Time: 20 minutes | Cook Time: 55 minutes

Nutritional Info:
Calories: 584, Fat: 24 g, Protein: 38 g, Carb: 60 g

Ingredients:

1/3 cup plain dry breadcrumbs
½ teaspoon paprika
3 ½ cups low fat milk, divided
2 cups low fat cottage cheese
4 cups extra sharp cheddar cheese
¼ teaspoon nutmeg powder
¼ teaspoon ground pepper
½ teaspoon salt or to taste
4 cups whole-wheat elbow pasta
2 teaspoons extra virgin olive oil
2 packages (16 ounces each) frozen spinach, thawed, pressed of excess moisture
6 tablespoons all purpose flour
Cooking spray

Directions:

1. Grease a large baking dish with cooking spray. Set aside.
2. Place a pot of water over medium heat. Bring to the boil. Add pasta and cook until the pasta is al dente. Once cooked, drain and set aside.
3. Meanwhile, add breadcrumbs, paprika and oil into a bowl and mix well.

4. Add 3 cups milk into a heavy bottomed saucepan. Place the saucepan over medium high heat. Bring to the boil.
5. Meanwhile mix together in a bowl, remaining milk and flour. Whisk until smooth.
6. Add the flour mixture into the boiling milk stirring constantly. Keep stirring until the sauce thickens. Turn off the heat and add cheddar cheese. Stir until it melts.
7. Add cottage cheese, nutmeg, salt and pepper. Stir until well combined.
8. Add pasta and stir. Transfer half the pasta mixture into the prepared baking dish.
9. Spread spinach on top. Spread the remaining half pasta over the spinach layer.
10. Sprinkle bread crumbs mixture all over the pasta layer. Cover with foil and place the dish in the refrigerator until use. To freeze, first cover the dish with plastic wrap and then with foil and place in the freezer until use. It can last for 2 days if refrigerated or for 3 months if frozen.
11. To use: Remove from the freezer and thaw in the refrigerator. Remove from the refrigerator an hour before baking.
12. Bake in a preheated oven 450° F for about 20 minutes or until golden brown in color.

Bacon Turkey Burger

Serving Size: 4 | Prep Time: 10 minutes | Cook Time: 35 minutes

Nutritional Info: For 1 burger
Calories: 354, Fat: 22 g, Protein: 40 g, Carb: 2.5 g

Ingredients:

1¼ pounds ground turkey
1 medium zucchini, shredded
2 cloves garlic, finely chopped
¼ teaspoon pepper or to taste
¼ pound bacon, cut into strips
1 small onion, finely chopped
½ teaspoon salt

To serve:
4 burger buns
Lettuce leaves, tomato slices or any other toppings of your choice

Directions:

1. Place a skillet over medium heat. Add bacon strips and cook until crisp.
2. Remove bacon with a slotted spoon and place on paper towels. When cool enough to handle, chop into fine pieces.
3. Retain 2 teaspoons of the fat in the skillet and discard the remaining.
4. Place the skillet back over medium heat. Add onion and garlic and sauté until translucent.

5. Remove from heat. Transfer into a bowl. Add rest of the ingredients into the bowl and mix well using your hands.
6. Divide the mixture into 4 equal portions and shape into patties.
7. Place a skillet or griddle over medium heat. Place the patties and cook for 3 minutes on each of the sides. Transfer into an airtight container. Refrigerate until use. It can last for 3 days. You can also place it in a freezer safe bag or container and freeze for up to 3 months.
8. Transfer the patties on a lined baking sheet. Thaw if frozen.
9. Bake in a preheated oven at 300°F for 15-20 minutes or until golden brown.
10. Serve in between buns. Place toppings of your choice and serve.

Note: Nutritional value of bun and toppings are not included.

Southwestern Cheddar Steak Fries

Serving Size: 8 | Prep Time: 20 minutes | Cook Time: 20 minutes

Nutritional Info:
Calories: 154, Fat: 5 g, Protein: 5 g, Carb: 22 g

Ingredients:

2 pounds red or Yukon gold potatoes, scrubbed, cut lengthwise into ¾ inch wedges
3 teaspoons smoked paprika
1 teaspoon garlic powder
Salt to taste
1 teaspoon ground cumin
2 tablespoons extra virgin olive oil
2/3 cup red bell pepper, finely chopped
2 ounces reduced fat sharp cheddar cheese, finely shredded
¼ cup fresh cilantro, finely chopped

Directions:

1. Line a baking sheet with foil. Place potatoes on it. Pour oil on it and toss well.
2. Mix together in a bowl, paprika, garlic powder and cumin. Sprinkle this mixture over the potatoes. Turn the potatoes and sprinkle on the other side too.
3. Transfer on to the prepared baking sheet. Spread it in a single layer. Bake in batches if required.
4. Bake in a preheated oven 425° F for about 20 minutes or until golden brown in color. It should be tender inside. Turn the potatoes half way through baking.

5. When done, remove from the oven. Cool and transfer into an airtight container. Refrigerate until use. It can last for 2-3 days.
6. To serve: Place potatoes on a baking sheet. Broil for a few minutes until crisp. Turn the potatoes and broil until crisp.
7. Mix together in a bowl, salt, pepper and cheese. Sprinkle it over the potatoes.
8. Bake for a few minutes until the cheese melts.
9. Garnish with cilantro and serve immediately.

Oven Baked Chicken Strips

Serving Size: 8 | Prep Time: 10 minutes | Cook Time: 25 minutes

Nutritional Info:
Calories: 147, Fat: 2.5 g, Protein: 6.1 g, Carb: 24.4 g

Ingredients:

4 chicken breasts cut into strips
2 teaspoons pepper powder or to taste
2 teaspoons salt or to taste
2 cups Italian style panko bread crumbs
2 cups flour
4 eggs

Directions:

1. Add flour, salt and pepper into a bowl. Mix well.
2. Add eggs into a second bowl. Beat well.
3. Add breadcrumbs into a third bowl.
4. First dredge chicken strips in flour. Next dip in egg. Shake to drop off excess egg. Finally dredge in breadcrumbs.
5. Place on a baking sheet that is lined with parchment paper.
6. Place the baking sheet in the freezer and freeze until it is hard.
7. Remove from the freezer and transfer into a freezer safe bag. Seal the bag and freeze until use.
8. To use: Remove from the freezer and place on a lined baking sheet.
9. Bake in a preheated oven 450° F for about 35-40 minutes or until golden brown in color. It should be tender inside and crisp outside. Flip sides half way through baking.

Mediterranean Chicken Quinoa Bowl

Serving Size: 8 | Prep Time: 5 minutes | Cook Time: 30 minutes

Nutritional Info:
Calories: 520, Fat: 27 g, Protein: 34 g, Carb: 31 g

Ingredients:

2 pounds chicken breasts, skinless, boneless
½ teaspoon pepper powder
½ teaspoon salt or to taste
½ cup almonds, slivered
2 small cloves garlic, crushed
1 teaspoon ground cumin
4 cups cooked quinoa
2 jars (7 ounces each) roasted red peppers, rinsed
½ cup extra virgin olive oil, divided
2 teaspoons paprika
½ teaspoon crushed red pepper (optional)

To serve:
½ cup kalamata olives, pitted, chopped
2 cups cucumber, chopped
¼ cup fresh parsley, chopped
½ cup red onions, finely chopped
½ cup feta cheese, crumbled

Directions:

1. Place the rack in the upper third of the oven. Place a sheet of aluminum foil on a baking sheet. Set aside.
2. Season chicken with salt and pepper and place on the baking sheet.

3. Broil until the chicken is tender at 450° F for 25-35 mins in pre heated oven. Remove the chicken from the oven and place on your work area. When cool enough to handle, slice the chicken or shred the chicken with a pair of forks.
4. Transfer chicken into an airtight container and refrigerate until use.
5. Also place cooked quinoa in another airtight container and refrigerate until use.
6. Add roasted red peppers, almonds, spices, garlic and ¼ cup oil into a blender and blend until smooth.
7. Transfer the sauce into an airtight container and refrigerate until use.
8. All the 3 containers can last in the refrigerator for 3 days.
9. To serve: Remove the containers from the refrigerator. Heat the ingredients in a microwave.
10. Add olives, red onions and remaining oil to quinoa and mix well.
11. Spoon the mixture into individual serving bowls. Divide and place cucumber and chicken on it. Drizzle red pepper sauce.
12. Top with feta cheese and parsley.

Buffalo Chicken Casserole

Serving Size: 4 | Prep Time: 15 minutes | Cook Time: 90 minutes

Nutritional Info:
Calories: 441, Fat: 12 g, Protein: 37 g, Carb: 47 g

Ingredients:

6 ounces whole-wheat elbow pasta
3 small carrots, sliced
1 medium onion, chopped
1 pound chicken breast, skinless, boneless, trimmed cut into 1 inch cubes
2 cups low fat milk
2 ½ tablespoons hot sauce or to taste
1 tablespoon canola oil
3 small stalks celery, sliced
½ tablespoon garlic, minced
2½ tablespoons cornstarch
Salt to taste
2 ounces blue cheese, crumbled

Directions:

1. Cook the pasta according to the instructions on the package but for 4 minutes lesser than that mentioned on the package. Drain and rinse and set aside.
2. Place a skillet over medium heat. Add oil. When the oil is heated, add carrots, onion, celery and garlic and sauté until the vegetables are slightly soft.
3. Add chicken and sauté for 6-7 minutes. It should not remain pink.

4. Add cornstarch and milk into a bowl and whisk. Pour it into the skillet stirring simultaneously. Add salt and bring to the boil. Stir frequently. Simmer until thick. Turn off the heat.
5. Add hot sauce and stir. Transfer the cooked pasta into a baking dish. Pour the chicken along with sauce over the pasta. Sprinkle blue cheese all over the dish.
6. Cover with foil and refrigerate until use. It can last for a day.
7. To freeze, first cover the dish with plastic wrap and then with foil and place in the freezer until use. It can last for 2 days if refrigerated or for 3 months if frozen.
8. To use: Remove from the freezer and thaw in the refrigerator. Remove from the refrigerator an hour before baking.
9. Bake in a preheated oven 400° F for about 45 minutes. Remove from the oven and serve after 10 minutes.

Smoky Beef Stew

Serving Size: 4 | Prep Time: 1 minutes | Cook Time: 120 minutes

Nutritional Info:
Calories: 341, Fat: 12 g, Protein: 42 g, Carb: 18 g

Ingredients:

1 pounds stewing beef, chopped into chunks
1 can (28 ounces) chopped tomatoes
1 can (14 ounces) butterbeans, drained, rinsed
1 medium onion, chopped
1 teaspoon sweet paprika
1 teaspoon ground cumin
1 teaspoon mild chili powder
1 tablespoon caster sugar
1 tablespoon red or white vinegar

Directions:

1. Add all the ingredients except beans in a casserole dish. Mix well. Cover with foil.
2. Bake in a preheated oven 320° F for about 2 hours. Add beans and stir. Bake for another 20-30 minutes or until beef is cooked. Remove from the oven and cool completely.
3. Transfer into freezer safe bags and freeze until use.
4. To use: Thaw in the refrigerator. Heat in a microwave or pan and serve.

Spicy Smoky Sweet Chili

Serving Size: 12 | Prep Time: 10 minutes | Cook Time: 60 minutes

Nutritional Info:
Calories: 354, Fat: 6 g, Protein: g, Carb: 42.9 g

Ingredients:

2 pounds ground beef
4 cloves garlic, minced
2 cans (29 ounces each) tomato sauce
2 cans (15 ounces each), black beans, drained
2 cans (15 ounces each) vegetarian baked beans
1 teaspoon onion powder
2 tablespoons chili powder or to taste
2 teaspoons smoky paprika
1 teaspoon garlic powder
1 teaspoon ground cumin
½ teaspoon cayenne pepper or to taste
2 large shallots or 1 large onion, chopped
Salt to taste
Pepper to taste
2-4 heaping tablespoons brown sugar
For toppings (optional): Use any as much as required
Green onion, thinly sliced
Sour cream
Cheddar cheese, shredded
Tortilla chips

Directions:

1. Place a large skillet over medium high heat. Add beef, shallots, salt, pepper and garlic and sauté until beef turns brown.
2. Add rest of the ingredients and stir.
3. Lower heat and cover with a lid. Simmer for about 30-40 minutes. Taste and adjust the sugar and seasonings if necessary.
4. When done, cool completely. Transfer into an airtight container or freezer safe bags and seal. Freeze or refrigerate until use. It can last for 2-3 days in the refrigerator and for 3 months if frozen.
5. To use: Thaw in the refrigerator. Heat in a microwave or pan and serve with the toppings of your choice.

Steak Burritos

Serving Size: 8 | Prep Time: 10 minutes | Cook Time: 30 minutes

Nutritional Info:
Calories: 472, Fat: 16 g, Protein: 31 g, Carb: 49 g

Ingredients:

1 cup prepared fresh salsa
½ cup instant brown rice
24 ounces strip streak, trimmed, sliced thinly crosswise
2 tablespoons canola oil
1 cup sharp cheddar cheese, shredded
¼ cup fresh cilantro, chopped
1 cup water
2 cans (15 ounces each) black beans, rinsed
Pepper to taste
Salt to taste
8 whole-wheat tortillas (8 inches each)
½ cup prepared guacamole

Directions:

1. Place a saucepan over medium heat. Add water and salsa and bring to the boil. Add rice and stir.
2. Lower heat and cover with a lid. Simmer for 5-7 minutes. Add beans and simmer without covering until rice is cooked. Stir a couple of times while it is cooking. Remove from heat and cool completely. Transfer into an airtight container and refrigerate until use. It can last for 2-3 days.
3. Meanwhile, season steak with pepper.

4. Place a large skillet over medium high heat. Add oil. When the oil is heated, add steak and cook until brown.
5. Remove from heat and cool completely. Transfer into an airtight container and refrigerate until use. It can last for 2-3 days.
6. To use: Heat the rice and steak. Warm tortillas according to the instructions on the package.
7. Spread the tortillas on your work area. Divide and place the steak among the tortillas. Divide and sprinkle cheese over it. Divide and spoon the rice, guacamole and cilantro.
8. Roll and serve.

Sole en Papillotte

Serving Size: 8 | Prep Time: 10 minutes | Cook Time: 15 minutes

Nutritional Info:
Calories: 201, Fat: 11 g, Protein: 22 g, Carb: 4 g

Ingredients:

8 sole fillets (4-6 ounces each)
1 teaspoon freshly ground pepper or to taste
4 tablespoons extra virgin olive oil
2 pints grape tomatoes, halved
1 teaspoon kosher salt or taste
4 cloves garlic, minced
¼ cup fresh basil, sliced
4 scallions, thinly sliced

Directions:

1. Cut 8 square sheets of parchment paper of 12 inches each. Fold each sheet of paper in halves and open it again.
2. Place a fillet on one side of the creased paper. Sprinkle salt, pepper and garlic. Drizzle oil. Place basil, tomatoes and scallions over fillet. Fold the other half of the paper over it and fold the edges to seal. Place on a large baking sheet.
3. Place the baking sheet in the refrigerator until use. It can last for a day.
4. To use: Bake in a preheated oven 400° F for about 15 minutes or until golden.
5. Place the packets on individual serving plates. Unwrap using a knife and serve.

Quick Shrimp Enchilada Bake

Serving Size: 4 | Prep Time: 10 minutes | Cook Time: 25 minutes

Nutritional Info:
Calories: 291, Fat: 6 g, Protein: 24 g, Carb: 36 g

Ingredients:

½ pound shrimp, peeled, deveined, tails discarded, diced
1 can (4 ounces) chopped green chilies with its liquid
6 corn tortillas
½ cup low fat Mexican style blend or Monterey Jack of cheddar cheese, shredded
Lime wedges to serve
½ cup frozen corn, thawed
1 cup canned green enchilada sauce or green salsa, divided
7½ ounces canned nonfat refried beans
¼ cup fresh cilantro, chopped
Cooking spray

Directions:

1. Grease a glass baking dish with cooking spray. Set aside.
2. Add corn, shrimp, chilies and ¼ cup enchilada sauce into a microwave safe bowl. Cover and heat in a microwave for about 1-2 minutes.
3. Spread about 2-3 tablespoons of enchilada sauce on the bottom of the prepared baking dish. Place 3 tortillas in the dish by overlapping it.
4. Spoon the refried beans all over the tortillas. Spread the shrimp mixture on it. Lay 3 more tortillas on it. Spread the remaining

sauce over the tortillas. Cover the dish with foil and refrigerate until use. It can last for a day.
5. To use: Remove the dish from the refrigerator an hour before baking.
6. Bake in a preheated oven 400° F for about 15 minutes. Sprinkle cheese on top and bake for another 5 minutes. Sprinkle cilantro and serve with lemon wedges.

Skillet Tuna Noodle Casserole

Serving Size: 3 | Prep Time: 10 minutes | Cook Time: 40 minutes

Nutritional Info:
Calories: 401, Fat: 8 g, Protein: 32 g, Carb: 46 g

Ingredients:

4 ounces whole-wheat egg noodles
1 small onion, finely chopped
¼ teaspoon salt
3 tablespoons all-purpose flour
¼ teaspoon freshly ground pepper or to taste
½ cup frozen peas, thawed
¼ cup coarse dry whole-wheat breadcrumbs
½ tablespoon extra virgin olive oil
4 ounces mushrooms, sliced
¼ cup dry white
1 ½ cups nonfat milk
6 ounces canned chunk light tuna, drained
½ cup Parmesan cheese, finely grated, divided

Directions:

1. Cook noodles according to the instructions on the package until al dente. Drain and rinse in cold water. Drain and set aside.
2. Place the rack of the oven in the upper third of the oven.
3. Place an ovenproof skillet over medium high heat. Add oil. When the oil is heated, add onion, mushroom and salt and cook until tender.

4. Add wine and stir. Simmer until dry. Sprinkle flour and mix well. Pour milk and stir constantly until it thickens. Add pepper, tuna, peas and half the Parmesan cheese and stir.
5. Stir until well combined. Add noodles and fold gently. Cover the skillet with foil and refrigerate until use. It can last for a day.
6. To use: Sprinkle breadcrumbs and remaining Parmesan cheese over the noodles. Cover the dish with foil
7. Bake in a preheated oven 400° F for about 15 minutes. Uncover and broil for few minutes until the top is golden brown.

Middle Eastern Lamb Stew

Serving Size: 4 | Prep Time: 10 minutes | Cook Time: 90-120 minutes

Nutritional Info:
Calories: 253, Fat: 14 g, Protein: 19 g, Carb: 12 g

Ingredients:

¾ pound lamb stew meat, boneless
2 teaspoons ground cumin
1/8 teaspoon cayenne pepper
Freshly ground pepper to taste
14 ounces canned diced tomatoes
2 cloves garlic, minced
3 ounces baby spinach to serve
½ tablespoon olive oil or canola oil
½ tablespoon ground coriander
¼ teaspoon salt or to taste
1 medium onion, chopped
6 tablespoons low sodium chicken broth
8 ounces canned chickpeas, drained, rinsed

Directions:

1. Mix together in a bowl, oil, cumin, coriander, cayenne, pepper and salt. Rub this mixture over the lamb.
2. Place a skillet over medium heat. Add broth, tomatoes and garlic and bring to the boil.
3. Add lamb and onions and stir. Lower heat. Cover with a lid. Simmer for 1 ½ -2 hours or until tender. Discard any fat that is floating on the top.

4. Add ¼ cup chickpeas into a bowl and mash it. Add into the skillet along with the remaining chickpeas. Simmer for 5-10 minutes. Remove from heat and cool completely.
5. Transfer into an airtight container and refrigerate until use. It can last for 2 days. You can also transfer into freezer safe bags and freeze for 4 months.
6. To use: Thaw the frozen stew in the refrigerator. Remove from the refrigerator an hour before serving. Transfer the contents into a saucepan. Add spinach. Heat thoroughly until the spinach wilts.

Conclusion

Once again, thank you for choosing this book.

Up until now, you might have thought meal planning was a big hassle and it could take a lot of your time. I hope that you are pleasantly surprised by how easy it is to prep for your meals and how it can, in fact, save a lot of your time. As someone who has been meal prepping for over 5 years, I urge you to take it slow at the beginning without overwhelming yourself so that you can experience all the fun in the process.

Try buying the freshest and organic ingredients from the local farmer's market. They are more flavorful and add a great taste to your dishes. The recipes mentioned in this book are extremely simple and can be tweaked to your convenience. I have tried to use the most basic ingredients and easy cooking methods to make your life simpler.

I wish to know what you think about this book. Feel free to send in your honest comments as I am looking forward to your constructive feedback on what you hope to see in subsequent books.

Made in the USA
Middletown, DE
08 February 2019